Eleanor Clarke Slagle

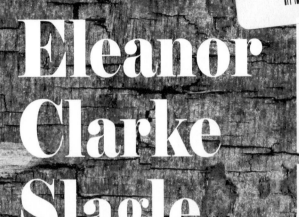

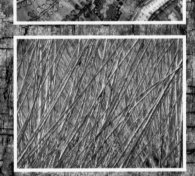

Mother of Occupational Therapy

Lori T. Andersen

ELEANOR CLARKE SLAGLE
Mother of Occupational Therapy

Lori T. Andersen, EdD, OTR/L, FAOTA

Cover Photos
Photographs on the cover represent occupational therapy products and materials. Patients engaged in basket weaving and rug making for the therapeutic benefit and economic benefit from sale of products. The willow branches represent the activity of growing and harvesting willow for use in making baskets and willow furniture. Eleanor Clarke Slagle had patients, as part of their therapy, plant, grow, and harvest willow for use in making products. This was a way to obtain materials for treatment at minimal expense, a cost effective measure for limited budgets.

Photo credits: Background—Anne Nygård@polarmermaid; Baskets—Hans Braxmeier; Rug/Tapestry—Lida Sahafzadeh@designedbylida; and Willow Branches—Hans Braxmeier.

Printed in the United States of America

Last digit is print number 10 9 8 7 6 5 4 3 2 1

DEDICATION

This book is dedicated to "Aunt Peggie."

Copies of letters sent by John Davenport Clarke to his sister Eleanor Clarke Slagle, which were found in the Research Library at the Fenimore Art Museum and at the Wilma West Library in the Archive of the American Occupational Therapy Association, often began with the salutation "Dear Aunt Peggie." In a personal email communication to me, Mrs. Slagle's grandniece confirmed that members of the Clarke family who knew Mrs. Slagle well addressed her as Aunt Peggie. So, to honor Mrs. Slagle and her family and in hopes that through this book we might get to know her better personally as well as professionally, this book is dedicated to Aunt Peggie.

Contents

ACKNOWLEDGMENTS

Writing this book was possible because of the support, guidance, and assistance of friends, colleagues, and a number of organizations. I am extremely grateful to all of you who helped me realize my dream to honor and memorialize the life of Eleanor Clarke Slagle.

My sincere appreciation goes to the following friends and colleagues:

Dr. Carol Niman Reed, my friend, colleague, and mentor, provided support and encouragement through the whole process of researching and writing the book. Dr. Reed reviewed numerous drafts, offering valuable suggestions and feedback to improve the organization and clarity of the manuscript.

Dr. Barbara A. Schell, an experienced book editor having edited several editions of *Willard and Spackman's Occupational Therapy,* reviewed the manuscript and offered constructive feedback to improve the organization, flow, and clarity. Dr. Schell also graciously agreed to write the Foreword.

Dr. Barbara L. Kornblau, a prolific writer and my friend, colleague, and mentor, provided support and encouragement, reviewed various aspects of the manuscript, and offered suggestions to improve the clarity of the writing.

Dr. Alma Abdel-Moty, my friend and colleague, reviewed the manuscript and offered helpful feedback to improve the organization and flow.

Judy Stewart Vidal, President of the Hobart Historical Society, encouraged me to write this book and inspired me to continue even when the goal seemed out of reach.

James G. (Jim) Meagley, who with the support of the Hobart Historical Society, compiled the book *A Look Back at Hobart, NY on the 125th Anniversary of the Village Incorporation, 1888-2013,* provided new information and clarification about locations in Hobart significant to Eleanor Clarke Slagle and her family.

Dr. Kathlyn "Kitty" Reed, PhD, OTR, FAOTA, MLIS, my colleague with whom I co-authored the book *The History of Occupational Therapy: The First Century,* shared her knowledge of occupational therapy history.

Many thanks to the Fenimore Art Museum, the Hobart Historical Society, the Delaware County Historical Society, and the American Occupational Therapy Association for giving permission to reprint photos from their respective archives; and to Erik Hinckley for giving permission to reprint his photo of Charles B. Clarke.

Thank you to the staff at the Florida Gulf Coast University library who were determined to obtain several "hard to find" archival journal articles, newsletter articles, and government reports for my research.

Thank you to Lauren Biddle Plummer (laurenplummer@comcast.net), a publishing professional, for editing, typesetting, and creating the cover design for the book.

And finally, thank you to John Bond, President of Riverwinds Consulting (www.riverwindsconsulting.com), who guided me through the publication process.

ABOUT THE AUTHOR

Lori T. Andersen, EdD, OTR/L, FAOTA received her Bachelor of Science degree in Rehabilitation Services from Springfield College in Springfield, Massachusetts; her Master of Science degree in Occupational Therapy from the Virginia Commonwealth University in Richmond, Virginia; and her Doctorate in Education from Nova Southeastern University in Fort Lauderdale, Florida. She is the author of several journal articles, book chapters, online continuing education courses, and presentations related to occupational therapy practice, professional issues, and professional education. In 2003, she was named a Fellow of the American Occupational Therapy Association for her contributions to the profession. After more than 15 years in clinical practice and more than 20 years in academia, she is now enjoying retirement, pursuing such passions as traveling, researching the history of occupational therapy, and writing. In recent years, she co-authored *The History of Occupational Therapy: The First Century* (2017), served as a consulting editor for and contributor to the Centennial Edition of *Willard and Spackman's Occupational Therapy* (2018), and wrote this book, *Eleanor Clarke Slagle: Mother of Occupational Therapy* (2022).

PREFACE

As a young girl, I enjoyed reading biographies and learning about people's lives. While doing research for the book *The History of Occupational Therapy: The First Century,* a book that I co-authored with Kitty Reed, I was fascinated by the people that gave the profession of occupational therapy its start and wanted to learn more about them. Mrs. Slagle was the most well-known of the six founders of the American Occupational Therapy Association, but in spite of her high profile no comprehensive study of her life and activities has been published. In fact, little was known about her early life and information about her professional life is scattered in articles and reports published several years ago. Wanting to learn more about Mrs. Slagle's life, I started to do more in-depth research using academic, archival, and genealogical resources.

For me, this type of research is, in part, about the thrill of the hunt and the joy in finding interesting facts and details and then putting the puzzle pieces together. Part of my research involved travel, something which I also enjoy. My travel included research trips to the Wilma West Library in Bethesda, Maryland where the American Occupational Therapy Association Archives are held (including correspondence between the founders) and a trip to the Research Library at the Fenimore Art Museum in Cooperstown, New York. The Research Library in Cooperstown holds the John Davenport Clarke (brother of Mrs. Slagle) papers and family photos. Additionally, I took three trips to Delaware County, New York to visit the village of Hobart and the Hobart Historical Society, the Delaware County Historical Association, and the Delaware County Court House.

At the Hobart Historical Society I found the handwritten minutes of meetings of the Hobart Woman's Civic Club that described the meetings in which Mrs. Slagle gave talks about her work. At the Delaware County Historical Society I found the handwritten minutes of meetings of the Grand Army of the Republic (GAR) when Mrs. Slagle's father, William J. Clark, was serving as Acting Adjutant and had recorded the minutes. At the Delaware County Court House in Delhi I found probate papers and property records. In Hobart, Mrs. Slagle's hometown, I was able to walk the streets where she walked, and I was able to see the locations where she was born, where she was married, and where she is buried.

As Mrs. Slagle left little in terms of personal papers, much of the information and evidence provided in this book comes from census records, church records, minutes of various associations and organizations, historical accounts in books and atlases, military and veterans records, government reports, marriage and divorce records, school records, probate papers, telephone and business directories, resumes, letters, old photographs, and other archival records and newspaper articles. Some of these records and documents were obtained through my research trips and some from searches of records available on the internet. All attempts were made to gather best evidence of family relationships, history, and activities; however, some evidence is more reliable than other evidence. Sources are provided in the reference citations to enable future researchers to weigh the evidence. It is my hope that future researchers will be able to confirm or correct information provided in this book as more evidence is found.

I learned a great deal about Mrs. Slagle's personal and professional life and her many contributions to the occupational therapy profession. Mrs. Slagle has always been held in high esteem by those in the occupational therapy profession, including me; but through my research it became very clear why she is so deserving of this admiration and respect. With this book I hope to keep her spirit and memory alive and hope to instill in others a greater understanding and appreciation for all she has done.

Foreword

Occasionally, you learn something about a colleague that reveals a whole new side of the person. Such was the case when Dr. Lori Andersen and I served on the same occupational therapy faculty at Brenau University in Gainesville, GA. Dr. Andersen was hired based on her experience in teaching students how to provide occupational therapy to individuals with physical disabilities. During lunchtime conversations I became aware of her interest in collecting occupational therapy historical artifacts. Soon after, I enlisted her as a guest lecturer on the history of the profession in the Foundations of Occupational Therapy course that I taught. Dr. Andersen brought in a treasure trove of historical items, along with a fount of knowledge about the founders of the American Occupational Therapy Association. Dr. Andersen's recognition as an authority on occupational therapy history has grown by leaps and bounds in the years since. In 2017 she, along with co-author Dr. Kathlyn Reed, published *The History of Occupational Therapy: The First Century*. Following that, I asked her to serve as a consulting editor for our new special feature "Centennial Notes" in the 13th edition of *Willard and Spackman's Occupational Therapy*, which I edited along with Dr. Glen Gillen. This text was published soon after the 100th anniversary of the profession. Dr. Andersen wrote and/or edited over 70 short pieces highlighting focused aspects of the profession's history.

I was thrilled to learn that Dr. Andersen was working on a book dedicated to Eleanor Clarke Slagle. Mrs. Slagle is one of the first founders of occupational therapy that students learn about in school. Occupational therapy professionals are regularly reminded of her at the American Occupational Therapy Association Annual Conference, where an award in her honor is a highlight of the recognition ceremonies. The Eleanor Clarke Slagle Lectureship was established as a memorial to Eleanor Clarke Slagle, one of the outstanding pioneers in the profession of occupational therapy, and recognizes an occupational therapy practitioner who has made substantial and lasting scholarly contributions to the profession. Award winners have a full year to prepare a scholarly lecture, and over time the "Slagle lectures" have themselves become important benchmarks in occupational therapy history.

Despite Eleanor Clarke Slagle's name recognition, very few individuals fully understand her background or the many contributions she made to occupational therapy and health care in the 20th century. Dr. Andersen's extensive and well-documented research brings to life Mrs. Slagle's extraordinary professional life. Mrs. Slagle operationalized the theoretical ideas of other founders, organized programs, innovated the actual therapy process, obtained funds to support these programs, and developed educational standards to assure that generations of therapists lived up the high ideals of the founders. In addition, Dr. Andersen synthesizes the scarcer, but equally intriguing information that hints at Mrs. Slagle's personal and family life and their role in motivating her life work.

The great gift that Dr. Andersen provides to the reader is the opportunity to really get to know Mrs. Slagle, both personally and professionally. This biography is of interest to a wide audience beyond those in the occupational therapy profession, such as those interested in the history of medicine, the history of the New York State Department of Mental Hygiene, and the history of Delaware County, New York. Finally, the biography is an important contribution to the slowly developing documentation of the contributions of women leaders in the first half of the 20th century.

Barbara A. Schell, PhD, OT/L, FAOTA
Professor Emerita, School of Occupational Therapy, Brenau University
Co-Owner, Schell Consulting, Athens, Georgia

A NOTABLE WOMAN
OF DELAWARE COUNTY,
NEW YORK

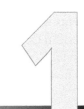

> *"Do not go where the path may lead,*
> *go instead where there is no path and leave a trail."*
> —Ralph Waldo Emerson

Eleanor Clarke Slagle was "a handsome woman, with large blue eyes and soft grey hair, just over 5 feet, 6 inches in height." Her soft, pleasant voice belied the power she held in her professional positions (Cromwell, 1977, p. 647). In childhood, she was known as Ella May Clark. As she reached her adult years, she went by the name Eleanor, although family and good friends would still call her Ella. When she entered professional life, she was addressed as Mrs. Slagle, a title commonly used for married women, and in her case, a title also used out of respect for her professional status. "A woman of strong personality, she possessed broad vision, charm, dignity, and a presence which commanded admiration and respect" (American Occupational Therapy Association, 1967, p. 292). In her professional roles, she was a demanding woman, yet one of culture, tact, a pleasing personality, and an extraordinary devotion to work on behalf of the occupational therapy profession (Cromwell, 1977).

With her sense of civic responsibility and interest in helping those with mental illness through the therapeutic use of occupation, she become a major force behind the development and expansion of occupational therapy in the United States and around the world. As one of the founders of the National Society for the Promotion of Occupational Therapy (NSPOT), later renamed the American Occupational Therapy Association (AOTA), she became an ambassador for occupational therapy. A charismatic personality, she was sought after by national and international groups to speak on her work in occupational therapy and to provide advice on establishing clinical and educational occupational therapy programs. According to Dr. Adolf Meyer, the renowned psychiatrist with whom Mrs. Slagle had worked, she was "the personification of occupational therapy" (Editorial Comment, 1942, p. 797).

Eleanor Clarke Slagle was a woman influenced by the times she lived in and a woman who, in turn, influenced the times. She was married at the age of 23 in 1894 and separated 16 years later in 1910, at a time when the role of women in society was changing. More women were entering the workforce, often working in jobs that promoted social responsibility. Mrs. Slagle was one of these women. Born in 1870, she was in her early 40s when she became interested in the therapeutic use of occupations to improve the quality of life of patients with mental illness, in her mid-forties when she became one of the founders of the American Occupational Therapy Association, and in her early 50s when the New York State Hospital Commission tapped her to direct all the occupational therapy departments in the state hospital system.

THE PROGRESSIVE ERA

The Progressive Era of the 20th century was the start of a new age in which science, education, and technology were highly valued, embraced, and used to support efforts to facilitate reform. With the start of this new era, many women (especially from the elite middle class) felt an obligation and duty to work for social reforms to improve the quality of life for people and communities. To this end, these women became involved in these movements that advocated for social reforms to promote quality of life for all in society. It was during this time that a confluence of movements helped shape and stimulate the growth and development of the new profession of occupational therapy. These movements included the Progressive Movement, the Arts and Crafts Movement, the Settlement House Movement, the Mental Hygiene Movement, and the resurgence of moral treatment in mental institutions.

The Progressive Movement sought to address the problems generated by the Industrial Revolution by promoting social justice and political reforms. The Industrial Revolution of the 19th century, a major turning point in history, is credited with improving the standard of living for society with positive changes such as improved manufacturing processes. Goods were mass-produced in factories, making them available to a more people. Jobs opened up in the new factories and offered many new employment opportunities. But in spite of the positive changes, the Industrial Revolution also generated some negative consequences—poor work conditions, low wages, child labor, and corruption. The Progressive Movement pushed for better work conditions, higher wages, restrictions on child labor, and an end to corruption in government and industry.

The Arts and Crafts Movement also started as a reaction to the Industrial Revolution by those who believed that mass production of goods, judged to be shoddy and of lesser quality than handcrafted goods, contributed to decline in standards, moral values, and quality of life. As a push-back to mass production, arts and craft societies formed in a number of cities to preserve individual creativity and the contributions of craftsmen. These societies embraced the idea that the use of one's hands in the process of making handcrafted goods helped to integrate the mind and body, provided intrinsic satisfaction, and as a result, improved quality of life (Andersen & Reed, 2017, p. 9).

The Settlement House Movement started in the United States in the late 1880s to address the problem of poverty in crowded immigrant neighborhoods and to help immigrants adapt to life in the United States. Immigrants were often looked on with suspicion as they had different values, customs, habits, rituals, religions, languages, and dress. Many of these foreign-born people were admitted to insane asylums because of these differences and difficulty adapting to their new home in the United States (Bockoven, 1963, p. 24; Luchins, 1988). By helping immigrants adapt, settlement houses helped them avoid admission to insane asylums. Hull House in Chicago, one of the best known settlement houses in the United States, provided organized educational programs to teach work skills to immigrants. Hull House also provided social and recreational activities and served as a neighborhood center where people of different sociocultural backgrounds could gather to exchange ideas and to learn about each other's cultures and backgrounds. The mission of settlement houses soon expanded to mirror the ideals of the Progressive Movement, working to promote social and political reforms. To achieve these goals, settlement houses also functioned as research centers, gathering information to influence social policy with a focus on such issues as public health, children's welfare, workplace safety, and consumer protection (Andersen & Reed, 2017, pp. 10-11).

Clifford W. Beers' autobiographical book, *A Mind that Found Itself*, spurred the Mental Hygiene Movement in the early 1900s. After suffering a mental breakdown, Mr. Beers was admitted to a number of insane asylums for treatment. His autobiography revealed the horrendous conditions in these asylums and subsequently started a national conversation to improve care for patients through better living conditions and individualized care in institutions. The National Committee for Mental Hygiene and a number of affiliated State Societies of Mental Hygiene started as a result of this conversation. The missions of these societies focused on facilitating change through the education of physicians and the public. The Mental Hygiene Movement was in alignment with the use of moral treatment in improving care of patients with mental illness (Andersen & Reed, 2017, p. 19).

The moral treatment philosophy, which originated in the 18th century in Europe, considered mental illness to be caused by the stresses of life. As such, treatment focused on providing humane living conditions in comfortable living environments with plenty of fresh air and light. Additionally, participation in occupation was recognized as beneficial to the well-being of patients, so rather than keeping patients chained or confined and left idle, participation in structured daily routines and occupations, including work, leisure, and exercise activities, was part of patients' treatment. During the early part of the Progressive Era, many institutions serving people with mental illness, including the New York State Hospital Commission, embraced the philosophy of moral treatment and started to recognize the value of therapeutic use of occupations and the new profession of occupational therapy.

The objectives of these Progressive Era Movements, to improve quality of life for all people in society, were embraced by many organizations in the early 20th century, including the New York State Hospital Commission. Seeking to improve and expand programs and services to enhance the quality of life for their patients, the New York State Hospital Commission hoped to recruit and hire Eleanor Clarke Slagle.

Note: The spelling of Clark (Clarke) varies in different documents and newspaper articles. The inconsistencies may be due to changes in how the family spelled their surname at different times in history or to misspellings of their surname. While today the "Clarke" version is the acceptable version, in this book, the spelling of Clark/Clarke will be used interchangeably depending on the time in history and/or cited source material.

A Prominent Position

In November of 1919, at the 20th New York State Conference of Charities and Correction, Dr. Charles W. Pilgrim, Chairperson of the New York State Hospital Commission, presided over a session in which Mrs. Slagle gave a presentation on the occupation therapy services that she supervised in the state of Illinois. At the conclusion of her talk, Dr. Pilgrim stated, "… I was particularly glad to hear her speak to us as 'home folks,' because we may be able to offer her sufficient inducements to get her to transfer efforts to this State." (New York State Conference of Charities and Correction, 1919, p. 129).

A few years later, on December 8, 1921 at a quarterly meeting of the State Hospital Commission, Mrs. Slagle read her paper on *Training of Aides for Mental Patients* (The State Hospital Quarterly, 1922a). In introducing Mrs. Slagle, the presiding chairperson, Dr. Charles W. Pilgrim, still remained hopeful that the Commission could hire Mrs. Slagle stating,

> We are exceptionally fortunate today in having with us one who has probably given more attention to the work of occupational therapy than anybody else in the country. It has been my hope during the past three or four years that we might impress upon the Legislature the importance of this subject and to induce them to give us an appropriation sufficient to enable us to avail ourselves of Mrs. Slagle's splendid abilities. I have not given it up yet. I hope the time may come when we can have someone like Mrs. Slagle to take charge of all our occupational therapy. (The State Hospital Quarterly, 1922a, p. 240)

A State Commission in Lunacy had been established in 1894 by the New York Constitution to oversee institutions that cared for those with mental illness (New York State, 1894). This commission was renamed the New York State Hospital Commission in 1912 (State Hospital Commission, 1913). Consistent with the focus of Progressive Movements of the early 20th century, to improve patient care for those with mental illness, the New York State Hospital Commission was actively working to obtain state funding to improve programs for patient care. Specifically, the commission wanted to develop an occupational therapy program and hire someone to oversee the program.

In 1922, the New York State Legislature made a special appropriation of $13,700 to develop the occupational therapy programs in state hospitals and to hire a director of occupational therapy. Mrs. Slagle was the choice of the state hospital commissioners, but first she needed to pass a competitive civil service examination that included both oral and written sections (Slagle, 1936; State Hospital Commission, 1923a; 1923b). Mrs. Slagle qualified for the position through the examination, was selected from a pool of five candidates (four men and one woman), and was officially appointed director of occupational therapy by the State Hospital Commission on July 1, 1922 (Slagle, 1936; State Hospital Commission, 1924, p. 3). Dr. Horatio Pollock announced her appointment at the 6th Annual Meeting of the American Occupational Therapy Association stating, "… we have been fortunate in securing the services of Mrs. Slagle who is now Director of Occupational Therapy in the New York State Hospitals for mental diseases, and we expect, in the course of a year or two, to put New York more decidedly on the map than it has been heretofore" (AOTA, 1923, pp. 321-322).

Like many women of that time period, Mrs. Slagle did not hold a job during her marriage and, like many women of that time period, she did not have a college education that would have prepared her for this prominent position. However, she did have a basic education and her life experiences growing up in Delaware County, New York shaped her values, beliefs, work ethic, commitment to service, and also developed her skills and abilities. Separated and then divorced in her 40s, she had the need and desire to pursue a career. Through these life experiences, she was prepared to succeed in this high-powered professional role.

The Influences on the Life of Ella May Clark

"We carry, inside us, people who came before us."
—Liam Callanan

Mrs. Slagle was undoubtedly influenced and shaped by the history and times of the area where she grew up; her neighbors; the personalities, values, beliefs, experiences, and work ethics of her immediate and extended families; as well as her deceased ancestors whose life stories she most likely heard. Some of these family members were leaders, some were adventuresome, some had a curious nature and the desire to learn about the world, and some were drawn to a life of service to others. Some of these family members had illnesses and injuries that affected their daily lives. Their experiences might have influenced Mrs. Slagle to pursue a career in a health care field.

Delaware County History

Mrs. Slagle grew up in the close-knit communities of Hobart and Delhi in Delaware County, New York where everyone knew each other, worked together, played together, and were always willing to lend a helping hand. Many of the residents who lived in these villages during the time Mrs. Slagle was growing up have descendants who still live there today.

The Clark(e) and Davenport families initially arrived in the area now known as Delaware County, New York toward the end of the 1700s and quickly became solid citizens of their communities. Situated in the Catskills Mountains in the south central part of New York that borders the northeast corner of Pennsylvania, Delaware County is a combination of rugged terrain and rolling hills (Figure 1-1). The Mohawk tribe, part of the Iroquois Confederation, inhabited the area in the 1700s. In the second half of the 1700s, a small number of European settlers started to move in. Most were Scotch-Irish pioneers who were filled with hope of a new life in a new world. Their dreams were put on hold when the Mohawks aligned with the British during Revolutionary War, attacking settlements and putting the new settlers' lives in danger. Many left the area concerned for their safety. Some returned after the war ended and more new settlers followed, increasing the population of the new communities (Duerden & LaFever, 2016, p. 7; Meagley, 2014, pp. 11-13; Munsell, 1880, pp. 50-51). These industrious settlers were driven by their dreams, values, beliefs, and customs to build a new life and new communities in an area full of natural resources and beauty.

With the end of the war and birth of the new country, and with continued development of settlements, the governmental structures and areas gradually evolved. County, town, and village borders were designated, but as more settlements developed, borders changed. One of these border changes occurred on March 10, 1797, when an act of the New York State Legislature formed Delaware County by merging parts of Ulster County and Otsego County. The towns of Davenport, Harpersfield, and the village of Hobart were

Figure 1-1. Location of Delaware County within New York State.

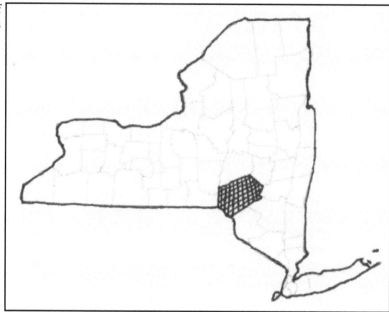

Figure 1-2. Map of Delaware County with towns.

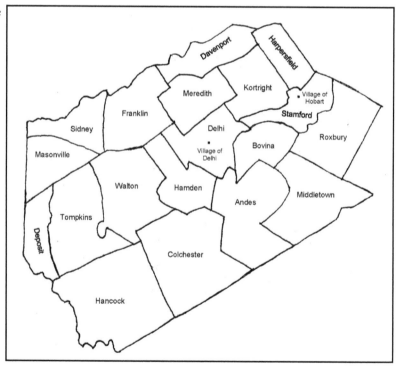

established in the northeast corner of Delaware County. Hobart, where Eleanor was born, was first known as Tinkertown, then Waterville, and finally Hobart (Figure 1-2). The village was renamed Hobart in 1828 when a village post office was about to be established. As there already was another Waterville post office in New York State, and there couldn't be

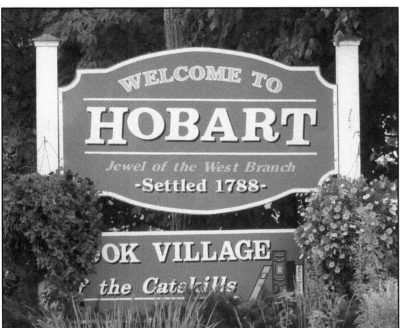

two, the name was changed to Hobart in honor of Episcopal Bishop John Henry Hobart, Third Bishop of the Episcopal Diocese of New York State (Meagley, 2014, pp. 17, 19, 20; Munsell, 1880, p. 301; Publicity Committee, 1913). Since the 1880s, Hobart's population has ranged from 400 to 600 inhabitants (Meagley, 2014, p. 16). Sitting on the West Branch of the Delaware River, Hobart, known as the Jewel of the West Branch, is now home to the Hobart Book Village (Figure 1-3).

Gristmills, lumbering, saw mills, dairy farming, butter making, harvesting maple sap, and making maple sugar were among the early industries in Delaware County (Munsell, 1880, p. 155; Murray, 1898, pp. 106-110). Transportation methods of the time were quite different from today. To move around the northeast corner of Delaware County, the people of Delaware County (including the Clarks and Davenports) relied on stage coach, horse drawn wagon, horse and buggy, horse-drawn sleighs in winter, horseback riding, walking, and then train starting in the mid-1870s to mid-1880s when rail service came to the county.

In the late 1800s and early 1900s, a tourist industry developed as the green rolling hills and cool mountain air in the summer and the trees ablaze with colors in the fall enticed tourists to the area (Duerden & LaFever, 2016, p. 8; Publicity Committee, 1913) (Figure 1-4). Cottages and boarding houses opened and large hotels were built to accommodate the tourists. In July of 1900, Mr. and Mrs. R. E. Slagle of Chicago (Eleanor and Robert, her husband at time) were listed among the tourists traveling to a hotel in Hobart to enjoy the pure air of the Catskills in the summer months ("Shades of the Catskills", 1900). The tourist industry thrived until World War II, when tourism began to decline. Some hotels decayed and were torn down, while some were lost to fire. The once popular tourist season became part of a bygone era.

Figure 1-4. Sightseeing in Hobart, New York circa 1907. (Reprinted with permission from the Hobart Historical Society, Hobart, New York.)

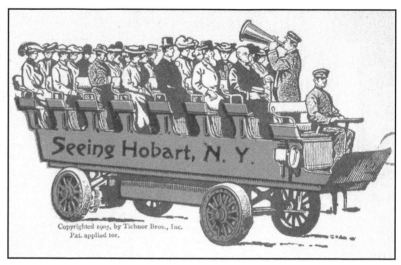

Seeing Hobart, N. Y.

Copyrighted 1907, by Tichnor Bros., Inc.
Pat. applied for.

THE CLARK(E) FAMILY OF HARPERSFIELD AND HOBART, NEW YORK

This story of the Clark family starts with Robert Clark and Julia (Beardsley) Clark, the *paternal grandparents* of Eleanor Clarke Slagle lived in Harpersfield, New York, in Delaware County. Robert was of Scotch-Irish heritage. Robert had six children in 11 years with his wife Julia (Clarke, 1933, June 5; U.S. Census, 1850; 1880a). The fifth child, William J. Clark, was Eleanor Clarke Slagle's father (see Appendix A). In the mid-1850s, the Clark family moved to Hobart, New York, to a house at the present day location of 284 Main Street in the village (Meagley, 2014, p. 93). The Clarks became a fixture in Hobart, with members of the family living in the Clark family homestead from the mid-1850s until 1906 when Frances Clark, the last Clark to live in the house, passed away.

On the evening of January 2, 1862, tragedy struck the Clark family when Robert Clark *(grandfather)*, the patriarch of the Clark family, walked the quarter mile to Scutt's Hotel in the village to enjoy the evening with friends and neighbors. A drunk patron became disorderly. Mr. Scutt, the landlord, requested Robert's help to eject the disorderly patron when the man grabbed Robert and threw him to the ground. Robert hit his head on the sidewalk, fracturing his skull. He died six hours later ("A Man Killed in Hobart", 1862; "Man Killed at Hobart,"1862). The site of this unfortunate incident, Scutt's Hotel, survives today with a new name, the Hobart Inn (Figures 1-5 and 1-6). Robert's widow, Julia Clark, continued to live in the Clark Family home on Main Street in Hobart until her death in 1889 ("Mrs. Julia E. Clark *[sic]*", 1889). She is buried with other members of the Clarke family in Locust Hill Cemetery.

The first child of Robert and Julia, John Clark *(uncle)*, was born in 1831. John was a carpenter like his father (U.S. Census, 1850). A full 5 feet 11 inches tall with a dark complexion, brown hair, and gray eyes, he enlisted in the 72nd New York State Volunteer Infantry on

Note: *To help the reader, when discussing Eleanor Clarke Slagle's relatives, the person's relationship to Eleanor will be put in parentheses and italicized.*

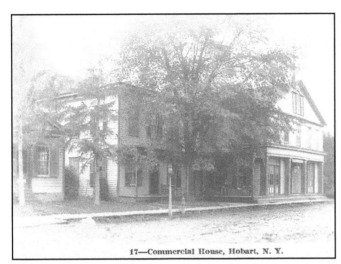

Figure 1-5. Old Postcard of the Hobart Inn, formerly Scutt's Hotel. (Reprinted with permission from the Hobart Historical Society, Hobart, New York.)

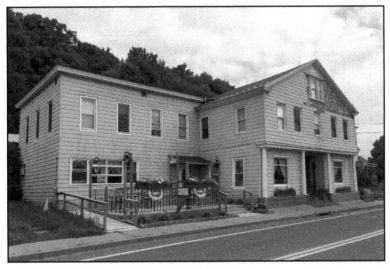

Figure 1-6. The Hobart Inn circa 2018. (© Lori T. Andersen. Reprinted with permission.)

June 4, 1861 at Delhi, New York. He mustered into Company I as a sergeant, serving under the command of General George McClellan through the Seven Days Battles near Richmond (June 25 to July 1, 1862), and was present when President Abraham Lincoln came to inspect the troops (Browne, 2012; Iron Brigader, 2016). Two weeks after Lincoln's visit, John was discharged for a disability, a hernia. He traveled home to Hobart where he enlisted in the 144th New York State Volunteer Infantry, the highly regarded regiment from the Delaware County area, in August 1862. He mustered into Company H of the 144th on September 27, 1862 as a 1st Lieutenant. John was promoted to full Captain on March 4, 1863, and served until he was discharged with the rest of the 144th on June 25, 1865 at Hilton Head, South Carolina.

After the war, John went home to live in the Clark family homestead in Hobart. He remained single, living with his mother and his sister Frances until 1886 when he moved to the Western Branch of the National Home for Disabled Volunteer Soldiers in Leavenworth, Kansas. He died there on March 6, 1900 and is buried in Leavenworth National Cemetery (Civil War Muster Roll Abstracts of New York State Volunteers, ca. 1861-1900a; Historical Register of National Homes for Disabled Volunteer Soldiers, 1866-1938; New York State

Division of Military and Naval Affairs, 2016, p. 754; Town Clerks' Registers of Men Who Served in the Civil War, ca. 1865-1867a; U.S., Burial Registers, Military Posts and National Cemeteries, 1862-1960) (Figure 1-7).

Born in Harpersfield in September 1832, Frances Clark *(aunt)* moved with her family to the Clarke Family House on Main Street in Hobart in the mid-1850s. She lived there until her death on Thursday, February 22, 1906. A teacher during her 20s (New York, State Census, 1855a), her reputation as a skilled dressmaker in her later years went far beyond the local area of Hobart. Occasionally when Frances traveled to New York City to see the new styles and to buy goods, she would take her niece Ella along to see the city ("Home and Vicinity", 1886; 1888).

Frances was an "omnivorous reader and a woman exceptionally well informed" ("Deaths of the Week", 1906). Her insatiable curiosity about the world continued

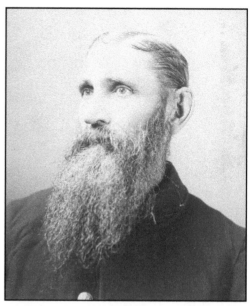

Figure 1-7. Captain John Clark, older brother of William J. Clark and uncle of Eleanor Clarke Slagle. (Reprinted with permission from the Research Library at the Fenimore Art Museum, Cooperstown, New York, John Davenport Clarke Papers, Coll. No. 12, Box 7.)

throughout her life. In September 1893, she and her niece Eleanor traveled to Rockford, Illinois in the Chicago area to visit a friend, Mrs. B. F. Lee. Eleanor and her aunt then traveled to Chicago on September 19, 1893 ("Purely Personal", 1893). Recognizing Aunt Frances' curious nature, they likely went there to attend the 1893 World's Columbian Exposition in Chicago (the Chicago World's Fair). There they would have seen and marveled at the power of electricity, used for the first time to light such a large area as the Chicago World's Fair. This display of technology spurred hopes of widespread use of electric power to light the world.

In 1901, her desire to learn more about the world inspired Frances to travel with a group of Hobart residents to the Pan-American Exposition in Buffalo, New York ("From the M-R Files", 1971). At this Exposition, the newly invented x-ray machine was on display; but perhaps the most notable event at this Exposition was the assassination of President William McKinley in early September, two weeks before Frances Clark and her friends attended the Exposition. The group viewed the spot in front of the Temple of Music where McKinley was assassinated.

A few years later Frances traveled to St. Louis to meet her niece Eleanor and to attend the 1904 St. Louis World's Fair. (Formally the name of the St. Louis World's Fair was the Louisiana Purchase Exposition in celebration of the centennial of the Louisiana Purchase.) The technology that debuted at this Exposition provided the public a view of the future, and included the first wireless telephone, the radiophone, and the personal automobile. Four years after the Exposition ended, Henry Ford began production of the Ford Model T—and in 1913 mass production of the Model T began, making automobiles more affordable for the general public.

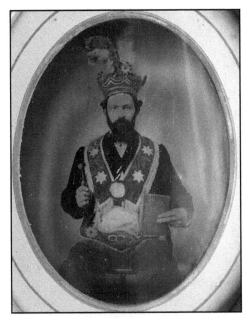

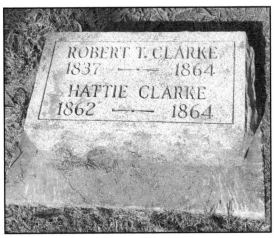

Figure 1-9. The gravestone of Robert T. Clarke and his infant daughter Hattie. Robert and Hattie died on the same day and were buried together. (© Lori T. Andersen. Reprinted with permission.)

Figure 1-8. Picture of Charles B. Clark, a member of the Independent Order of Odd Fellows (I.O.O.F.), dressed in his Odd Fellows garb, circa 1864. (Reprinted with permission from Erik S. Hinckley.)

Frances, who never married, was devoted to her niece, Eleanor Clarke Slagle, and her nephew, John Davenport Clark. When Eleanor and John's parents separated, Frances became their surrogate parent. Eleanor and John lived with their Aunt Frances off and on during this troubled time. Although Frances had other nieces and nephews, she left the bulk of her estate, including the Clarke Family House, to her favorite niece and nephew, Eleanor and John ("Deaths of the Week", 1906; Clark, 1906).

The second son, Charles B. Clark *(uncle)*, worked as a cooper in Hobart with William Beardsley before moving to Davenport and later the Albany area (Meagley, 2014, p. 331). Charles was a member of the Independent Order of Odd Fellows (I.O.O.F.), an organization whose mission is to help those in need including the elderly, youth, the sick, and to make the community a better place to live (Figure 1-8). He married Caroline Davenport *(aunt)* on June 19, 1866 ("Married", 1866). Charles and Caroline had several children, many of whom died in childhood. Charles moved his family to Albany near the end of the 1800s where he worked first as a farmer and then as a gardener (New York, State Census, 1905; U.S. Census Bureau, 1900a).

The third son, Robert T. Clark *(uncle)*, a farm laborer, (U.S. Census, 1860), married Harriet Ballagh on February 7, 1860 in Harpersfield ("Married", 1860a). Sadly, the Clark family suffered another tragedy in 1864 when Robert T. Clark was mortally wounded in a street fight in Hobart. He was stabbed with a butcher knife by a man named John Mitchell (New York, State Census, 1865). He died on August 31, 1864, the same day that his infant daughter Hattie died. Robert and Hattie were buried in the same grave in Locust Hill Cemetery ("The Hobart Stabbing Case", 1864) (Figure 1-9). Robert's assailant, John Mitchell, was tried and convicted of second degree manslaughter in February 1866, and sentenced to four years in Auburn prison in New York State for his crime. He was pardoned on May 19, 1869 and released from prison with all his civil rights restored (Executive Clemency and Pardon Application Ledgers and Correspondence, 1849-1919; "Trial for Murder", 1866).

The fourth son, William J. Clark, Eleanor Clarke Slagle's father, was born in Harpersfield on June 27, 1840. He led an interesting life that brought him to many regions of the United States. In his teenage years, he worked as a laborer in the farm fields in the town of Colchester in Delaware County (New York, State Census, 1855b). In 1858, he went to the Kansas territory known as Bloody Kansas, where he lived with a family named Baysinger. There he is reported to have served with the abolitionist John Brown in the Kansas-Missouri Border wars. In the summer of 1859, William was badly wounded near Fort Scott, Kansas—shot by horse thieves. Soon after, he contracted malaria and, in a twist of fate, the illness made it impossible for him to travel with John Brown to Harpers Ferry where Brown's famous raid took place in October 1859 (Kansas Territory Census, 1859; "With John Brown", n.d.).

William returned home to Hobart in 1860. With the call for volunteers to serve in the Union Army, William enlisted in the 144th New York State Volunteer Infantry. Physically imposing at 6 feet tall with black eyes, black hair, and a dark complexion, William was a natural leader. He mustered into the 144th on September 27th as a Corporal in Company H and was promoted

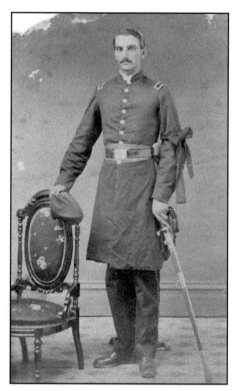

Figure 1-10. William J. Clark, Second Lieutenant in the 144th NYS Volunteer Infantry. (Reprinted with permission from the H. Fletcher Davidson Library Archives, Delaware County Historical Association. Delhi, New York.)

to Sergeant on May 1, 1863. He was promoted again to 1st Sergeant on May 15, 1864 and to 2nd Lieutenant on November 28, 1864 (Civil War Muster Roll Abstracts of New York State Volunteers, ca. 1861-1900b; Town Clerks' Registers of Men Who Served in the Civil War, ca. 1865–1867b) (Figure 1-10).

After spending time in Washington, DC; Maryland; and Virginia, the 144th New York State Volunteer Infantry traveled further south to engage the Confederate Army in South Carolina. In September 1863, while encamped near Charleston, South Carolina, William was shot in the neck by a rebel sharpshooter during a skirmish at James Island. While the bullet barely missed his spinal cord ("The Last of John Brown's Raiders", n.d.), the wound caused him to thereafter suffer from neuralgia. Because of this neck wound he was granted a government disability pension of $8.00 a month in January 1875 (List of Pensioners on the Roll, 1883, p. 85). The extent of this disability and the specific symptoms that he had are not known, however, it seems that this disability did not severely limit his life activities as after the war as he worked in strenuous jobs: a cooper, a sheriff, and a builder of houses and bridges. He also participated in fire department musters, athletic contests after the war which required strength, speed, and agility.

William was discharged with the others in the 144th on June 25, 1865 at Hilton Head, South Carolina. The 144th returned to Delhi, New York where all the soldiers were officially

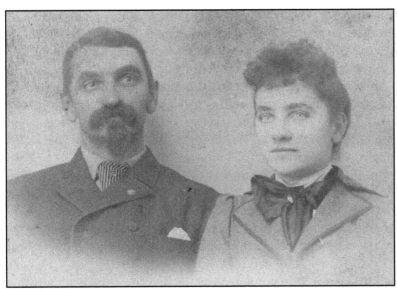

Figure 1-11. William J. Clark and woman presumed to be Emma, his wife. The inscription on the back of the photo reads, "William Clarke + wife"; however, it is not known who wrote the inscription or when. (Reprinted with permission from the Research Library at the Fenimore Art Museum, Cooperstown, New York, John Davenport Clarke Papers, Coll. No. 12, Box 7.)

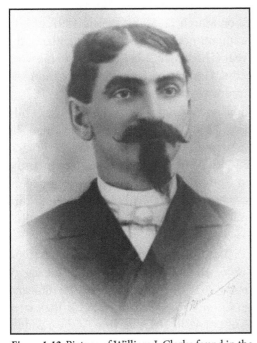

Figure 1-12. Picture of William J. Clarke found in the Hobart Historical Society Building, site of the old St. Andrew's Masonic Lodge, No. 289. (Reprinted with permission from the Hobart Historical Society, Hobart, New York.)

mustered out on September 27, 1865, three years to the day after they had mustered in (Civil War Muster Roll Abstracts of New York State Volunteers, ca. 1861-1900b; Town Clerks' Registers of Men Who Served in the Civil War, ca. 1865-1867b).

William returned to Hobart to live in the Clark family homestead, and like his brother Charles, he worked as a cooper making tubs, churns, and firkins, which were small wooden buckets with lids. The churns were used to make butter, while firkins were used to store butter (Beers, 1869; U.S. Census, 1870a). On July 17, 1867 he married Emma J. Davenport of Davenport, New York, who was the sister of Caroline Davenport—his brother Charles' wife (Figure 1-11). In the 1870s, while living in Hobart with his wife and family, William became a member of St. Andrew's Masonic Lodge, No. 289, F. & A. M. He served as the Master from 1874 through 1876, and he remained a member of that lodge until his death in 1897. In 1889, while William was still a member and living in the area, the St. Andrew's Masonic Lodge built a new Masonic Temple on Cornell Street in Hobart. This building was used by the Masons until 1996 when they surrendered their charter and ownership of the building was transferred to the Hobart Historical Society (Heinmiller, 2010, p. 27) (Figure 1-12).

At the end of 1876, William was elected sheriff of Delaware County on the Republican ticket by a substantial majority. In early 1877, he moved his family to Delhi, New York (the county seat) so he could serve his three-year term. When his term as sheriff ended, he continued to live in Delhi. Although he did not actively engage in a regular business, he did build some houses on Clinton Street in Delhi and was also hired to some repair bridges in the Delhi area. William also took time to travel, starting with an extended trip with his wife to visit Indiana, Nebraska, Kansas, and Wisconsin, among other states ("Commissioner's Report", 1887; "Commissioner's Report", 1888; " Delhi progress in a year", 1884; "The Last of John Brown's Raiders", n.d.).

A founding member of the Delhi Fire Department on April 11, 1860 (Welch, 1897, p. 12), he continued his interest in fire service through the 1880s, serving with the Delhi Fire Department, the Clinton Fire Department in Hobart, and with Clark's Independent Hose Company ("The Oxford Fire Parade", 1880). Actively involved in the fire department, he enjoyed organizing and participating in fire department parades, tournaments, musters, bean bakes, and clambakes.

William J. Clark was also active in the Grand Army of the Republic (G.A.R.), a post-war organization of Union Soldiers. A charter member of the England Post, No. 142, the Delhi, New York chapter of the G.A.R. that was organized on March 11, 1880 (Welch, 1897, pp. 30-31; G.A.R. England Post No. 142, 1880, p. 1), he was unanimously elected Commander of the No. 142, England Post in 1886 and served for one year (Hitchcock, 1885). Similar to his work with the fire department, he participated by organizing Decoration Day (Memorial Day) and Fourth of July events, as well as numerous G.A.R. reunions and encampments.

Addie Clark *(aunt)* (also known as Adelia, Adda, and Adelaide) was the youngest child of Robert and Julia Clark, born in 1842 (U.S. Census, 1850). She was 17 years old when she married Francis O. Richardson on July 12, 1860 ("Married", 1860b). At the age of 22, Francis Richardson (Find A Grave, 2017a), enlisted in the 144th New York State Volunteer Infantry. He served with John Clark and William J. Clark in Company H. Francis was discharged on May 18, 1864 due to a disability while at the military hospital on David's Island in New York Harbor ("144th Reg't N. Y. Volunteers from Delaware County," 1862; Civil War Muster Roll Abstracts of New York State Volunteers, ca. 1861-1900c).

Addie and Francis had one son, Charles W. C. Richardson, born on January 1, 1866 (Find A Grave, 2017b). When Francis died in October 1866, Addie became a widow at the age of 24, left alone to care for their infant son (Find A Grave, 2017a). Sometime between 1867 and 1869, Addie married William W. Burdick of Otsego County (U.S. Census, 1870b). They were only married a few years when William died at the age of 41 in 1873, leaving Addie a widow

Note: The evidence supporting Addie Clark Richardson's marriage to William W. Burdick is based on 1870 U.S. Census data that lists an Ada C. living with her husband Wm. W. Burdick and son Charles. The 1875 NYS Census and 1880 lists Adda Burdick as a widow living with her son Charles, consistent with information which indicates William W. Burdick died in 1873. The 1870 and 1880 Census data lists her son's name as "Charles," while the 1875 New York State Census data lists her son as "Charles Richardson." Charles' age is consistent with his birth year of 1866 in all these censuses, supporting the belief that "Charles" and "Charles Richardson" were the same person.

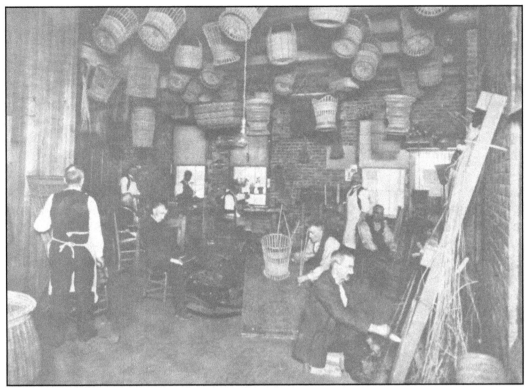

Figure 1-13. Patients making baskets, mats, and brushes at Willard State Hospital.

for the second time (Find A Grave, 2010). A two-time widow now, Addie worked as a dress-maker and a laundress to provide for herself and her young son (New York, State Census, 1875a; U.S. Census, 1880f).

In the 1880s, Addie married a widower, Isaac D. Gillespie of New Milford, Pennsylvania. She became a widow for the third time when he died in April 1895 ("Died", 1895). She worked as a servant for a time in Pennsylvania, then moved back to New York State (U.S. Census Bureau, 1900d; Williams, 1902, p. 326). In April 1902, she was hired by Willard State Hospital in Ovid, New York to work as an attendant. The hospital, first known as Willard Asylum for the Insane, opened in October 1869 for patients with mental illness. Attendants at this institution, following the philosophy of moral treatment, engaged patients in various occupations including craft activities, games, outdoor work activities, and other diversions and entertainment rather than keeping them locked up or chained (Gable, 2018) (Figure 1-13). Two years after she began her work at Willard State Hospital, Addie became seriously ill with pneumonia. She died on April 10, 1904 (Willard State Hospital, 1905, p. 23) and was buried in Glenwood Cemetery in Homer, New York with her first husband, Francis O. Richardson (Find A Grave, 2017c; "Homer", 1904).

THE DAVENPORT FAMILY OF DAVENPORT, NEW YORK

Emma Davenport *(Eleanor's mother)* was born on April 1, 1849 to John Davenport II and Catherine (nee Flansburgh) Davenport. Emma Davenport *(mother)*, who has been described by some as "frivolous" (DuVivier, 1976, p. 1), married William J. Clark on July 17, 1867 when she was 18 and he was 27. Caroline *(aunt)*, her older sister, had become the wife of William's older brother Charles in 1866.

John Davenport II *(maternal grandfather)* was the son of John Davenport I, a successful merchant, *(maternal great-grandfather)* and the Davenport's household servant, Betsy Williams. John Davenport I was the namesake of Davenport, New York; the town's first supervisor; and a descendant of the Reverend John Davenport of Stamford, Connecticut, an English Puritan clergyman whose vision helped found Yale University. Betsy Williams moved out of the Davenport household prior to giving birth to John Davenport II and was later known as Betsy Palmatier after her marriage to a Mr. Palmatier.

It is not clear whether Anna Davenport *(wife of Eleanor's maternal great-grandfather)* knew at the time that her husband fathered John II. When John I died in 1829, presumably of a stroke, he left the bulk of his estate to his son John II. His wife Anna contested the will, charging that John I was of unsound mind and memory when his will was written and signed. The case, tried in February 1830, garnered much interest in the county with 52 sworn witnesses testifying to the deceased's state of mind at the time he signed the will. The court found that John Davenport I was not of sound mind or memory at the time he executed the will, so the will was not admitted to probate (Briggs, 2004; Griswold, 2004a). However, it is possible that John Davenport II was eventually awarded part of his father's estate. In September 1830, at a time when women had no legal standing and could not serve as a guardian, Betsy Parmenter *[sic]* successfully petitioned the Surrogate Court to appoint James Ells of Harpersfield guardian to John Davenport II and his estate, properties, monies, and belongings until John turned 14 years of age (New York. Surrogate's Court [Delaware County], 1970).

In the early 1840s when he was 18 years old, John Davenport II *(maternal grandfather)* married Catherine Flansburgh *(grandmother)* (Griswold, 2004b). Catherine passed away in 1889. Two years later, on January 29, 1891, John II married Katherine Brown (Katie Brown) Davenport (Davenport, 1891) (see Appendix B).

John, a farmer, operated the family farm in Davenport until 1902. His sons engaged in a number of different occupations. James *(uncle)* was a cooper, and in later life, a hotel keeper and a laborer. John Jr. *(uncle)* worked as a painter, as well as other odd jobs. Lorin *(uncle)* was a jeweler, and Frank *(uncle)* was a paper hanger and a farm laborer. George *(uncle)* worked as a farm laborer and a carpenter. George died in 1892 at the age of age 37, suffering from tuberculosis (Davenport, 1892; New York, State Census, 1875b; U.S. Census, 1880b, 1880c, 1880d, 1880e, 1900b, 1900c).

While Eleanor likely had much more interaction with members of the extended Clark family since she lived closer to them, the physical distance between the Clark and Davenport families allowed them to get together using the various transportation methods of the time. Family gatherings with immediate and extended Clark and Davenport families were a significant part of Eleanor Clarke Slagle's early life. These gatherings, along with day-to-day interactions with family members, provided opportunities for Eleanor to learn life skills from family members and to hear the stories about her ancestors.

Sense of community, resilience, leadership ability, organizational ability, intellectual curiosity, a broad vision, and desire to serve and to help others (all characteristics in various members of the extended Clark and Davenport families) were characteristics that Eleanor also demonstrated. These characteristics, along with along with the attributes her professional colleagues identified in her: broad vision, charm, dignity, tact, a pleasing personality, a presence which commanded admiration and respect, and an extraordinary devotion to work on behalf of the occupational therapy profession, facilitated her success in her professional roles.

REFERENCES

144th Reg't N. Y. Volunteers from Delaware County. (1862, September 16). *Bloomville Mirror,* p. 2. Retrieved from www.fultonhistory.com

A man killed in Hobart. (1862, January 8). *Delaware Gazette,* p. 2. Retrieved from http://nyshistoricnewspapers. org/lccn/sn83030838/1862-01-08/ed-1/seq-2/

Andersen, L. T., & Reed, K. L. (2017). *The history of occupational therapy: The first century.* SLACK Incorporated.

American Occupational Therapy Association. (1967). Presidents of the American Occupational Therapy Association. *American Journal of Occupational Therapy, 21*(5), 290-298.

AOTA. (1923). The sixth annual meeting of the American Occupational Therapy Association, Fourth day, Morning session. *Archives of the American Occupational Therapy Association, 2*(4), 309-328.

Beers, F. W. (1869). Bovina, Hobart: Hobart business directory. In *Atlas of Delaware County New York 1869.*

Bockoven, J. S. (1963). *Moral treatment in American psychiatry.* Springer Publishing Company, Inc.

Briggs, M. S. (2004). *Chapter 3—Organization of the Town of Davenport. Davenport, Fact and Fancy.* Davenport Historical Society. Retrieved from http://www.dcnyhistory.org/Fact_Fancy/book/chap03.htm.

Browne, P. (2012, July 21). *McClellan's failure at Harrison's Landing.* Retrieved https://historicaldigression. com/2012/07/21/mcclellans-failure-at-harrisons-landing/

Civil War Muster Roll Abstracts of New York State Volunteers, United States Sharpshooters, and United States Colored Troops. (ca. 1861-1900a). *Record of John Clark.* Microfilm, 1185 rolls. New York State Archives, Albany, New York. Archive Collection #: 13775-83; Box #: 567; Roll #: 223 p. 311. Retrieved from www.ancestry.com

Civil War Muster Roll Abstracts of New York State Volunteers, United States Sharpshooters, and United States Colored Troops. (ca. 1861-1900b). *Record of William J. Clark.* Microfilm, 1185 rolls. New York State Archives, Albany, New York. Archive Collection #: 13775-83; Box #: 567; Roll #: 223 p. 318-319. Retrieved from www. ancestry.com

Civil War Muster Roll Abstracts of New York State Volunteers, United States Sharpshooters, and United States Colored Troops. (ca. 1861-1900c). *Record of Francis O. Richardson.* Microfilm, 1185 rolls. Archive Collection #: 13775-83; Box #: 569; Roll #: 225, p. 1464. New York State Archives, Albany, New York. Retrieved from www. ancestry.com

Clark, F. (1906). *Last will and testament of Frances Clark.* Records of the Surrogate's Court, County of Delaware, Delhi, New York.

Clarke, J. D. (1933, June 5). *Letter to American National Conference Against Racial Persecution in Germany.* Research Library at the Fenimore Art Museum, (Collection 12, Box 3, Folder 16), Cooperstown, NY.

Commissioner's report. (1887, February 9). *Delaware Gazette,* p. 2. Retrieved from http://nyshistoricnewspapers. org/lccn/sn83030838/1887-02-09/ed-1/seq-2/

Commissioner's report. (1888, February 15). *Delaware Gazette,* p. 2. Retrieved from http://nyshistoricnewspapers.org/lccn/sn83030838/1888-02-15/ed-1/seq-2/

Cromwell, F. S. (1977). Eleanor Clarke Slagle, the leader, the woman. *American Journal of Occupational Therapy, 31*(10), 645-648.

Davenport. (1892, July 12). *Stamford Mirror,* p. 1. Retrieved from www.fultonhistory.com

Davenport, C. (1891). *Diary of Clara Davenport.* H. Fletcher Davidson Library Archives, Delaware County Historical Association. Delhi, New York.

Deaths of the week. (1906, February 24). *Hobart Independent,* p. 1. Retrieved from www.fultonhistory.com

Delhi progress in a year. (1884, December 30). *Stamford Mirror.* Retrieved from www.fultonhistory.com

Died. (1895, April 12). Gillespie. *Montrose Democrat,* p. 3. Retrieved from www.newspapers.com

Duerden, T., & LaFever, R. (2016). *Images of America: Delaware County.* Arcadia Publishing.

DuVivier, P. T. (1976). *A congressman during hard times*. Unpublished manuscript–thesis. State University of New York College at Oneonta. Manuscript obtained from the Research Library at Fenimore Art Museum, Cooperstown, New York.

Editorial comment. (1942, December). Eleanor Clarke Slagle. *The Psychiatric Quarterly, 16*(4), 797-799.

Executive Clemency and Pardon Application Ledgers and Correspondence. (1849-1919). *Record of John Mitchell*. New York State Archives; Albany, NY, USA; Series Number: A0629; Volume: 4. Retrieved from www.ancestry.com

Find A Grave. (2010). *Memorial page for William W. Burdick*. Retrieved from https://www.findagrave.com/memorial/52437047/william-w-burdick

Find A Grave. (2017a). *Memorial page for Francis O. Richardson*. Retrieved from https://www.findagrave.com/memorial/182805612/francis-o-richardson

Find A Grave. (2017b). *Memorial page for Charles W. C. Richardson*. Retrieved from https://www.findagrave.com/memorial/182805633/charles-w_c_-richardson

Find A Grave. (2017c). *Memorial page for Adelaide Clarke Richardson*. Retrieved from https://www.findagrave.com/memorial/182805623/adelaide-richardson

From the M-R files: 70 years ago. (1971, September 29). *Stamford Mirror Recorder*, p. 2. Retrieved from www.fultonhistory.com

Gable, W. (2018). *The Willard Asylum for the insane*. Retrieved from https://www.co.seneca.ny.us/wp-content/uploads/2018/04/4-13-18-Willard-Asylum-full-history-ADA.pdf

G.A.R. England Post No. 142. (1880, March 11). *G.A.R. Book of minutes, No. 1, England Post No. 142*. H. Fletcher Davidson Library Archives, Delaware County Historical Association. Delhi, New York.

Griswold, J. (2004a). *John Davenport (I). Davenport Story: Additional materials for Davenport, Fact and Fancy*. Davenport Historical Society. Retrieved from http://www.dcnyhistory.org/Fact_Fancy/additional/davstory/ANCES/FG01/FG01_106.HTM

Griswold, J. (2004b). *John Davenport (II). Davenport Story: Additional materials for Davenport, Fact and Fancy*. Davenport Historical Society. Retrieved from http://www.dcnyhistory.org/Fact_Fancy/additional/davstory/ANCES/FG01/FG01_074.HTM

Heinmiller, G. L. (2010). *Craft Masonry in Delaware, New York*. Retrieved from http://www.omdhs.syracusemasons.com/

Historical Register of National Homes for Disabled Volunteer Soldiers. (1866-1938). *Record of John Clark*. National Archives Microfilm Publication M1749, 282 rolls; Records of the Department of Veterans Affairs, Record Group 15; National Archives, Washington, D.C. Retrieved from www.ancestry.com

Hitchcock, G. W. (1885, December 7). *Minutes—Annual meeting. Records of England Post G.A.R. No. 142*. Book no. 2, pp. 91-92. H. Fletcher Davidson Library Archives, Delaware County Historical Association. Delhi, New York.

Home and vicinity. (1886, October 14). Miss F. Clark went to New York, Tuesday... *Hobart Independent*, p. 3. Retrieved from www.fultonhistory.com

Home and vicinity. (1888, October 25). Miss F. Clark went to New York, Monday... *Hobart Independent*, p. 3. Retrieved from www.fultonhistory.com

Homer. (1904, April 14). The remains of Mrs. Addie C. Gillespie..., *Cortland Standard*, p. 8. Retrieved from www.fultonhistory.com

Iron Brigader. (2016, October 16). *The Berkeley Plantation's Harrison's Landing served as Union Army headquarters and encampment after the Seven Days Battles*. Retrieved from https://ironbrigader.com/2016/10/16/berkeley-plantations-harrisons-landing-served-union-army-headquarters-encampment-days-battles/

Kansas Territory Census. (1859). *Census of 1859, Township of Palmyra, County of Douglas, Kansas Territory, p. 13, line 20*. Retrieved from www.ancestry.com

List of pensioners on the roll. (1883). *List of pensioners on the roll, January 1, 1883, Vol. 2*. Government Printing Office.

Luchins, A. S. (1988). The rise and decline of the American asylum movement in the 19th century. *The Journal of Psychology: Interdisciplinary and Applied, 122*(5), 471-486.

Man killed at Hobart–Coroner's inquest–The evidence–Verdict of the jury. (1862, January 7). *Bloomville Mirror*, p. 1. Retrieved from www.fultonhistory.com

Married. (1860a, April 3). *Bloomville Mirror*, p. 3. Retrieved from www.fultonhistory.com

Married. (1860b, August 14). *Bloomville Mirror,* p. 3. Retrieved from www.fultonhistory.com

Married. (1866, July). *Delaware Republican.* Retrieved from www.fultonhistory.com

Meagley, J. G. (2014). *A look back at Hobart, NY on the 125th Anniversary of the Village Incorporation, 1888-2013.* Hobart Historical Society.

Mrs. Julia E. Clark *[sic],* widow of the late Robert Clark ... (1889, July 6). *Delaware Republican.* Retrieved from www.fultonhistory.com

Munsell, W. W. (1880). *History of Delaware County, N. Y. with illustrations, biographical sketches and portraits of some pioneers and prominent residents.* W. W. Munsell & Co.

Murray, D. (1898). *Delaware County, New York: History of the century, 1797-1897. Centennial celebration, June 9 and 10, 1897.* William Clark, Publisher.

New York, State Census. (1855a). *Harpersfield, County of Delaware.* Line 30 – 34, June 4, 1855, p. 2. FHL microfilm 832,847. Retrieved from www.familysearch.org

New York, State Census. (1855b). *E. D. 3, Colchester, County of Delaware. Line 41, Wm. J. Clark, June 21, 1855.* Microfilm. New York State Archives, Albany, New York. Retrieved from www.ancestry.com

New York, State Census. (1865). *Stamford, County of Delaware. Deaths occurring during the year ending June 1, 1865.* Line 10, Robert Clark, June 28, 1865, p. 44. Microfilm. New York State Archives, Albany, New York. Retrieved from www.ancestry.com

New York, State Census. (1875a). *Sherburne, County of Chenago, household of Ad*da Burdick. Lines 19 - 20. June 23, 1875, p. 14. Microfilm. New York State Archives, Albany, New York. Retrieved from www.ancestry.com

New York, State Census. (1875b). *E. D. 1, Davenport, County of Delaware, household of John Davenport.* Line 7-13, June 12, 1875. Microfilm. New York State Archives, Albany, New York. Retrieved from www.ancestry.com

New York, State Census. (1905). *City of Albany, County of Albany, household of Charles B. Clarke.* Lines 44 - 46. June 1, 1905, p. 12. New York State Archives, Albany, New York. Retrieved from www.ancestry.com

New York State. (1894). *Fourth Constitution of New York, 1894: Article VIII, Section 11.* Albany, NY: New York State. Retrieved from https://www.nycourts.gov/history/legal-history-new-york/documents/Publications_1894-NY-Constitution.pdf

New York State Conference of Charities and Correction. (1919). Fourth Session, Wednesday Afternoon, November 12, 1919 - Occupational therapy. In *Proceedings of the Twentieth New York State Conference of Charities and Correction* (pp. 121-135). Syracuse, NY: November 11-13, 1919.

New York State Division of Military and Naval Affairs. (2016). *72nd Infantry Regiment Civil War Unit Roster.* Retrieved from http://dmna.ny.gov/historic/reghist/civil/rosters/Infantry/72nd_Infantry_CW_Roster.pdf

New York. Surrogate's Court (Delaware County). (1970). *Matter of the guardianship of the person and estate of John Davenport. Of the Town of Davenport. Probate records, 1803-1930.* Salt Lake City, Utah: Filmed by the Genealogical Society of Utah. Retrieved from https://www.familysearch.org/ark:/61903/3:1:3QS7-L992-39XL-3?i=74&wc=Q759-JWP%3A213304401%2C221415001&cc=1920234

Publicity Committee. (1913). *Hobart-in-the Catskill Mountains, New York.* The Citizens' Association. Retrieved from www.hobarthistoricalsociety.org

Purely personal. (1893, September 20). *Morning Star* (Rockford IL), p. 8. Retrieved from www.genealogybank.com

Shades of the Catskills. (1900, July 7). *New York Herald,* section 4, p. 5. Retrieved from www.newspapers.com

Slagle, E. C. (1936). The past, present and future of occupational therapy in the State Department of Mental Hygiene. *Psychiatric Quarterly, 10*(1), 144-156.

State Hospital Commission. (1913). Title page. In *Twenty-fourth Annual Report of the State Hospital Committee.* J. B. Lyon Company, Printers.

State Hospital Commission. (1923a). Occupational therapy. In *Thirty-fourth Annual Report of the State Hospital Committee* (p. 36). J. B. Lyon Company, Printers.

State Hospital Commission. (1923b). The year in review. In *Thirty-fourth Annual Report of the State Hospital Committee* (p. 81). J. B. Lyon Company, Printers.

State Hospital Commission. (1924). Changes in the office force of the commission. In *Thirty-fifth Annual Report of the State Hospital Committee* (p. 3). J. B. Lyon Company, Printers.

The State Hospital Quarterly. (1922a, February). Minutes of the Quarterly Conference–December 8, 1921. *The State Hospital Quarterly, 7*(2), 226-241.

The Hobart stabbing case: Death of Clark. (1864, September 6). *Bloomville Mirror,* p. 2. Retrieved from www.fultonhistory.com

The last of John Brown's raiders. (n.d.). *Clipped newspaper article from Scrapbook 2, John Davenport Clark's papers.* Research Library at Fenimore Art Museum, Cooperstown, NY.

The Oxford fire parade. (1880, October 16). *Delaware Republican.* Retrieved from www.fultonhistory.com

Town Clerks' Registers of Men Who Served in the Civil War (ca. 1865–1867a). *Record of John Clark.* Microfilm publication, 37 rolls. New York State Archives. Albany, New York. Collection Number: (N-Ar)13774; Box Number: 16; Roll Number: 10. Retrieved from www.ancestry.com

Town Clerks' Registers of Men Who Served in the Civil War (ca. 1865–1867b). *Record of William J. Clark.* Microfilm publication, 37 rolls. New York State Archives. Albany, New York. Collection Number: (N-Ar)13774; Box Number: 16; Roll Number: 10. Retrieved from www.ancestry.com

Trial for murder. (1866, February 20). *Bloomville Mirror,* p. 2. Retrieved from www.fultonhistory.com

U.S., Burial Registers, Military Posts and National Cemeteries. (1862-1960). *Record of John Clark.* [database on-line]. Provo, UT, USA: Ancestry.com Operations, Inc., 2012. Retrieved from www.ancestry.com

U.S. Census. (1850). *Harpersfield, County of Delaware, State of New York, household of Robert Clark.* Lines 17-25, July 26, 1850, p. 345. Microfilm. Retrieved from www.familysearch.org

U.S. Census. (1860). *Harpersfield, County of Delaware, State of New York, household of Robert T. Clark.* Lines 7-8, July 26, 1860, p. 96. Microfilm. Retrieved from www.familysearch.org

U.S. Census Bureau. (1870a). *Stamford, County of Delaware, State of New York, household of William J. Clark.* Line 16, August 11, 1870, p. 2, Roll: M593_924; Page: 443B, Retrieved from www.ancestry.com

U.S. Census Bureau. (1870b). *Edmeston, County of Otsego, State of New York, household of Wm. W. Burdick.* Lines 35-37, July 18, 1870, p. 32. Roll: M593_1075; Page: 106B. Retrieved from www.ancestry.com

U.S. Census Bureau. (1880a). *Davenport, County of Delaware, State of New York, household of Alexander Clark.* Line 47, June 23, 1880, p. 35. Microfilm. Retrieved from www.familysearch.org

U.S. Census Bureau. (1880b). *Davenport, County of Delaware, State of New York, household of James Davenport.* Line 43, June 22, 1880, p. 33. Retrieved from www.ancestry.com

U.S. Census Bureau. (1880c). *Davenport, County of Delaware, State of New York, household of John Davenport.* Lines 13-16, June 26, 1880, p. 41. Retrieved from www.ancestry.com

U.S. Census Bureau. (1880d). *Davenport, County of Delaware, State of New York, household of John Davenport Jr.* Line 10, June 22, 1880, p. 33. Retrieved from www.ancestry.com

U.S. Census Bureau. (1880e). *Davenport, County of Delaware, State of New York, household of Lorin Davenport.* Line 29, June 22, 1880, p. 30. Retrieved from www.ancestry.com

U.S. Census Bureau. (1880f). *Norwich, County of Chenago, State of New York, household of Adda Burdick.* Lines 20-21, June 8, 1880, p. 18. Retrieved from www.ancestry.com

U.S. Census Bureau. (1900a). *Bethlehem township, County of Albany, State of New York, household of Chas. B. Clark.* Lines 20-24, June 8, 1900, Sheet No. 7. FHL microfilm 1241006. Retrieved from www.ancestry.com

U.S. Census Bureau. (1900b). *Davenport, County of Delaware, State of New York, household of Frank Davenport.* Line 2, June 9, 1900, Sheet No. 4. FHL microfilm 1241021. Retrieved from www.ancestry.com

U.S. Census Bureau. (1900c). *Davenport, County of Delaware, State of New York, household of James Davenport.* Line 17, June 13, 1900, Sheet No. 9. FHL microfilm 1241021. Retrieved from www.ancestry.com

U.S. Census Bureau. (1900d). *New Milford Borough, County of Susquehanna, State of Pennsylvania, Addie Gillespie in the household of Chas C. Pratt.* Line 23, June 13 & 14, 1900, p. 123. FHL microfilm 1241489. Retrieved from www.ancestry.com

Welch, E. L. (1897). Historical souvenir of Delhi, NY. *Grip's Valley Gazette.*

Willard State Hospital. (1905). *Thirty-sixth annual report of the Willard State Hospital to the State Commission in Lunacy for the year 1904.* J. B. Lyon Co., Printers.

Williams, J. E. (1902). *Williams' Broome County and Binghamton Directory City for 1902. Alphabetical directory. Address listing for Addie C. Gillespie,* p. 326. The Modern Press, Printers. Retrieved from www.ancestry.com

With John Brown. (n.d.). *Recollections of the hero of Harper's Ferry. Marion Martin in the Chicago Record.* Clipped newspaper article from Scrapbook 2, John Davenport Clark's papers, Research Library at Fenimore Art Museum, Cooperstown, NY.

The Early Life
of Ella May Clark

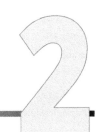

"Life is a lively process of becoming."
Douglas MacArthur

Ella May Clark was born to William J. Clark and Emma (nee Davenport) Clark in the small village of Hobart, New York in Delaware County on October 13, 1870 (Figures 2-1 to 2-3). She was their second child. Like her older brother John Davenport Clark (born on January 15, 1869), she was born in the Clark family homestead ("Happenings of Particular...", 1927; Meagley, 2014, p. 93) (see Appendix C) even though the family had purchased a house about 200 yards east of the Clark Family homestead in February 1869 (Delaware County Clerk, 1869; J. Meagley, personal communication, August 15, 2018) (see Appendix D). The Clark family homestead was most likely chosen for the location of Ella May's birth to allow William's mother Julia *(paternal grandmother)* and his sister Frances *(aunt)* to help Emma during childbirth and the early days after Ella's birth. Ella's first years were spent in the new Clark house overlooking the West Branch of the

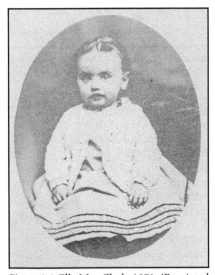

Figure 2-1. Ella May Clark, 1871. (Reprinted with permission from the Research Library at the Fenimore Art Museum, Cooperstown, New York, John Davenport Clarke Papers, Coll. No. 12, Box 7.)

Note: In this book, as a general rule of thumb, when referring to Eleanor Clarke Slagle, the name "Ella Clark" will be used from her birth through the early 1890s; the name "Eleanor Clark(e)" will used during the 1892 to 1894 time frame to concur with newspaper articles and documents from that time period; and the names "Eleanor Clarke Slagle" and "Mrs. Slagle" will be used for the time frame after her 1894 marriage to Robert E. Slagle.

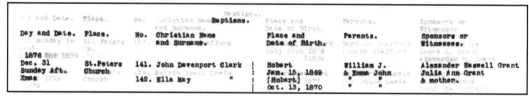

Day and Date.	Place.	No.	Christian Name and Surname.	Place and Date of Birth.	Parents.	Sponsors or Witnesses.
1876 Dec. 31 Sunday Aft. Xmas	St.Peters Church	141. 142.	John Davenport Clark Ella May "	Hobart Jan. 15, 1869 [Hobart] Oct. 13, 1870	William J. & Emma John " "	Alexander Haswell Grant Julia Ann Grant & mother.

Figure 2-2. Baptismal record of John Davenport Clark and Ella May Clark from St. Peter's Episcopal Church in Hobart, New York, transcribed by the New York Genealogical and Biographical Society in 1921 and edited by Royden Woodward Vosburgh (St. Peter's Episcopal Church [Hobart, NY], Vosburgh, R. W., & New York Genealogical and Biographical Society, 1921).

LOCATION.				NAME	RELATION.		PERSONAL DESCRIPTION.					
IN CITIES.		Number of dwelling-house, in the order of visitation.	Number of family, in the order of visitation.	of each person whose place of abode on June 1, 1900, was in this family. Enter surname first, then the given name and middle initial, if any. INCLUDE every person living on June 1, 1900. OMIT children born since June 1, 1900.	Relationship of each person to the head of the family.		DATE OF BIRTH.		Age at last birthday.	Whether single, married, widowed, or divorced.	Number of years married.	Mother of how many children.	Number of these children living.
Street.	House Number.					Color or race.	Sex.	Month.	Year.					
	1	2	3		4	5	6	7		8	9	10	11	12
35	292 92 279			Slagle, Robert E.	Head.	W.	M.	Oct.	1863	36	M.	6		
36				Eleanor M.	Wife.	W.	F.	Oct.	1870	29	M.	6	0	0

Figure 2-3. 1900 U.S. Census of Hyde Park Township, Cook County, Illinois, showing birth months and years of Robert E. and Eleanor M. Slagle.

Figure 2-4. The William J. and Emma Clark house stood at the location of this house at 431 West Main Street. The original Clark house no longer exists. The current house standing on the lot now was built in 1885, after the Clark family moved to Delhi (J. Meagley, personal communication). (© Lori T. Andersen. Reprinted with permission.)

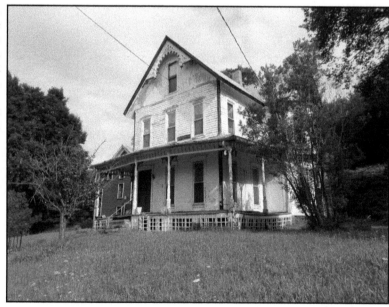

Delaware River (New York, State Census, 1875) (Figures 2-4 and 2-5). Due to the proximity of the Clark family homestead to William and Emma's house, in her early years Ella likely had frequent interaction with her grandmother Julia, her uncle John, and her Aunt Frances.

In the first six years of Ella's life, she lived in Hobart where her father worked as a cooper. He was elected sheriff of Delaware County, New York in November 1876. Soon after, William

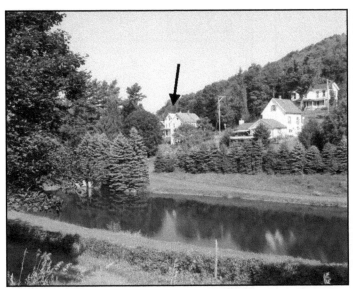

Figure 2-5. The arrow points to the location of the William J. and Emma Clark house at 431 West Main that overlooked the West Branch of the Delaware River. (© Lori T. Andersen. Reprinted with permission.)

moved the family to Delhi, the county seat, to serve his three-year term. Since the family had close ties to Hobart's civic and community life before moving to Delhi, Ella and her brother were baptized in the local church, St. Peter's Episcopal Church. The congregants attending that December 31, 1876 ceremony might have gotten a glimpse of Ella's indomitable spirit which would serve her well throughout her life. In a June 29, 1931 letter that John sent to his sister he writes, "Going to Hobart to-day for the 130th celebration of St. Peter's, where they had such a time baptizing you" (Clarke, 1931) (Figures 2-6 and 2-7).

Records documenting Ella Clark's early education are sketchy, incomplete, and, in some cases the dates of attendance are in conflict. A transcript from the Chicago School of Civics and Philanthropy (1911) documenting Eleanor Clarke Slagle's previous training, indicates that she attended the Delaware Academy in Delhi, New York for three years, although the dates of attendance are not recorded on the transcript. Most likely she attended Delaware Academy sometime between 1877 and 1885 when the Clarks lived in Delhi close to the Delaware Academy campus. From the 1850s until the late 1930s, the Delaware Academy campus was located on the present day site of the State University of New York Delhi (SUNY Delhi). In 1940, it was relocated to its present location on the old Sheldon Estate (Delaware Academy Central School District at Delhi, 2021; Welch, 1897, p. 20) (Figure 2-8).

William J. Clark and Emma Clark started having marital difficulties in the early 1880s, resulting in their separation in 1886. Shortly after the separation, Emma Clark left the home she shared with her husband William and their children and returned home to live with her father John Davenport in Davenport, New York. On July 1, 1889, Emma took up residence in Great Bend, Pennsylvania to establish and meet the residency requirements to file for divorce in Susquehanna County, Pennsylvania. In 1890, after meeting the one year residency requirement, Emma filed for divorce (Clark vs. Clark, 1890). The divorce was granted on January 28, 1891 and, as written in the divorce decree, it was "the answer to her prayers" (Clark vs. Clark, 1891). Emma then married William A. Happ on February 25, 1891, one month after her divorce was final ("Carthage", 1891; Pennsylvania, County Marriages [1885-1950], 2016; Susquehanna County, Commonwealth of Pennsylvania, 1891). Throughout the years they were married, Mr. Happ held assorted positions with various railroad companies.

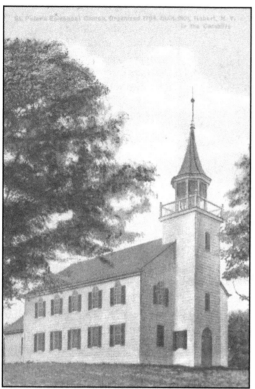

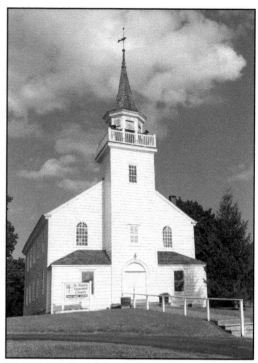

Figure 2-7. St. Peter's Episcopal Church circa 2017. (© Lori T. Andersen. Reprinted with permission.)

Figure 2-6. Old postcard of St. Peter's Episcopal Church, Hobart, New York. (Reprinted with permission from the Hobart Historical Society, Hobart, New York.)

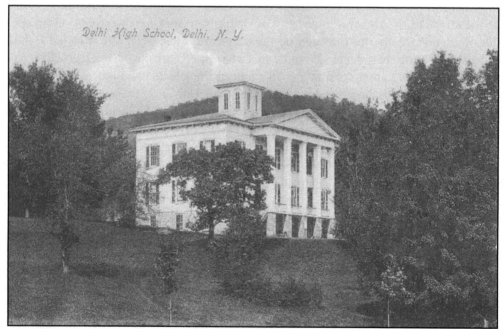

Figure 2-8. Old postcard of the old Delaware Academy in Delhi, New York. The site is now the home of the State University of New York (SUNY) at Delhi. (In Lori T. Andersen's collection. Printed with permission.)

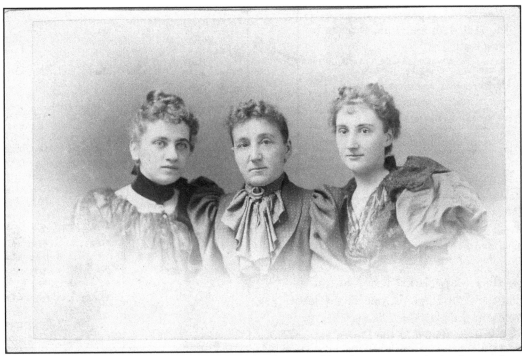

Figure 2-9. Ella May Clark (on left) circa mid-1880s. The identities of the other two women in the photograph are not known. (Reprinted with permission from the Research Library at the Fenimore Art Museum, Cooperstown, New York, John Davenport Clarke Papers, Coll. No. 12, Box 7.)

Railroad work was seasonal as more trains ran in the better weather during the tourist season in the spring, summer, and fall. Fewer trains ran during the inclement weather in the winter ("Being Pushed Along", 1895; "Carthage", 1888; "Glenfield", 1915a; "Town Tattle", 1905).

With the changes in the family situation, Ella and her brother John were sent away to school. She attended classes at the Claverack College/Hudson River Institute in New York State from 1885 to 1886 (Chicago School of Civics and Philanthropy, 1911; "Ella Clark and Jennie Middlemist...", 1885; "Miss Ella May Clark...", 1886) and in 1886 and 1887 she and her brother John were enrolled in classes at Starkey Seminary and College, a boarding school in Eddytown, New York ("Ex-Sheriff Clark…", 1886; "Miss Fannie Bordon, Miss Ella Clark…", 1886; "Miss Gussie Bowne…", 1887). It is unclear if either of them received any type of degree or certificate of completion from either of these educational institutions (Figure 2-9).

PERFORMING ARTIST AND FUNDRAISER

In her teenage years, Ella Clark was drawn to the performing arts, rehearsing with different community groups to present plays to the local townspeople. Most of the presentations served as fundraisers for the sponsoring community groups. In January 1885, the England Post, No. 142, Grand Army of the Republic in Delhi, New York, sponsored the play *Reward* to raise funds for the post (G.A.R. England Post No. 142., 1885, pp. 65-66). Ella Clark played the role of Kate Riley and her father, William J. Clark, played the role of George Hudson, a Virginian. This play was performed at the Opera House in Delhi on January 13, 14, 15, and 16, 1885 ("Reward will be Presented…", 1885) (Figure 2-10).

Reward will be presented here January 13th, 14th, 15th and 16th, with the following cast:

Fritz Stein, fresh from Faderland,   Charlie Collins.
Tom Markham, " True Blue," the Scout,
                                      J. M. Gordon.
Walter Greenwood, Southerner—Union,
                                      F. L. Norton.
George Hudson, a Virginian,   -   W. J. Clark.
Mr. Harris,   -   -   -   -   W. R. Whitney.
Sam Watson, who died for the flag,   H. J. Perkins.
Ike Smith, Hudson's pal,   -   G. W. Hitchcolk.
Jim Johnson, an innocent cause,   -   A. A. Raff.
Dick Osgood, a Union soldier,   -   C. F. Churchill.
Bob Winslow, Union Scout,   -   W. H. Douglass.
Officer of the Day,   -   -   -   J. D. Ferguson.
Grace Harris,   -   -   -   Miss Satie Sturges.
Kate Riley,   -   -   -   -   Miss Ella Clark.
Miss Mehitable,   -   -   Miss Emma Elliott.
Mrs. Harris,   -   -   -   Miss Lillie Cormack.
Goddess of Liberty,   -   Miss Emma Whitney.
        Scouts, Mountainers, Soldiers, Etc.

Figure 2-10. Cast of *Reward*—A newspaper clipping from the *Delaware Gazette*, January 7, 1885.

Ella May Clark's next role was as Phoebe Ann Hopkins, one of the lead roles, in the play *Uncle Rube*. This play was first presented at the Opera House in Delhi on November 15, 16, and 17, 1888 for the benefit of the Delhi Fire Department ("Home and Vicinity", 1888b) and then performed at the Hobart

" Uncle Rube."

Following is the cast of characters in the Drama, " Uncle Rube," to be produced under the auspices of the Hobart Fire Department, Jan. 17th, 18th and 19th:

Reuben Hopkins, Esq., of Perkinsville,
Vt., "who is trustee in our dees-
trick."   -   -   -   Mr. A. C. Sidman
Phœbe Ann Hopkins, his better two-
thirds,   -   -   Miss Ella May Clark
Betsey Hopkins,   -   Miss Millie MacNaught
Orrin Hopkins,   -   -   Mr. O. S. Faulkner
Widow Stebbins,   -   Miss Fannie B. Griffin
Avery Stebbins,   -   -   Mr. E. O. Grant
Augustus Clifton,   -   -   Mr. C. O. Rollins
Mrs. Meredith,   -   -   Miss Mae Tennant
Lucretia,   -   -   -   Miss M. M. Prentice
Alice Morton,   -   -   Miss M. S. Kennedy
Harry Harding,   -   Mr. G. K. MacNaught
Jim Taylor,   -   -   -   Mr. S. W. Rich
Bill Thompson,   -   Master Tom Kennedy
Officer Talbot,   -   -   Mr. C. H. King
John,   -   -   -   Mr. Percy Farrar
Newsboy,   -   -   Master Frank McNaught

Figure 2-11. Cast of *Uncle Rube*—A newspaper clipping from the *Hobart Independent,* January 10, 1889.

Village Hall on January 17, 18, and 19, 1889 under the auspices of Hobart Fire Department. Ella played the role of Phoebe Ann Hopkins in both these venues; however, when the play was performed in Hobart, the other roles were recast and played by Hobart residents ("Uncle Rube", 1889) (Figure 2-11). Miss Mae Tennant, one of the Hobart residents who played the role of Mrs. Meredith, was a childhood friend of Ella's—a friendship that continued into their adult years when they also developed a professional relationship through their connections to the Woman's Civic Club of Hobart.

Miss Ella Clark's talent for music was on display when she was selected as the pianist for the play *Esther: The Beautiful Queen*. A music course she completed, given by Professor Deyo in Poughkeepsie, New York ("Personals", 1889a), undoubtedly helped her with this performance. Professor Milo Deyo was a well-known concert pianist and director of the Poughkeepsie Piano School ("Milo Deyo Dies; Concert Pianist", 1925; R.V. LeRay Co., 1889, p. 111). This play was presented on March 4, 5, and 6, 1890 in Grant's Opera Hall in Hobart. Residents of the Hobart community comprised the large cast and chorus, including her friend Miss Mae Tennant who was a member of the chorus. Cost for a general ticket was 25 cents and a reserved seat was 35 cents ("Grant's Opera Hall", 1890) (Figures 2-12 to 2-14). Her participation in these community theatre presentations served to help Eleanor develop an ability and comfort presenting to groups both large and small, and taught her how to work with others to a successful end.

Her father's activities with the Masons, the G. A. R., and the fire departments instilled in Eleanor a sense of civic responsibility and service to others. Following in her father's footsteps, Eleanor supported some of these same civic organizations by participating in their fundraising activities. She assisted with the Masonic Fair held during the second week in

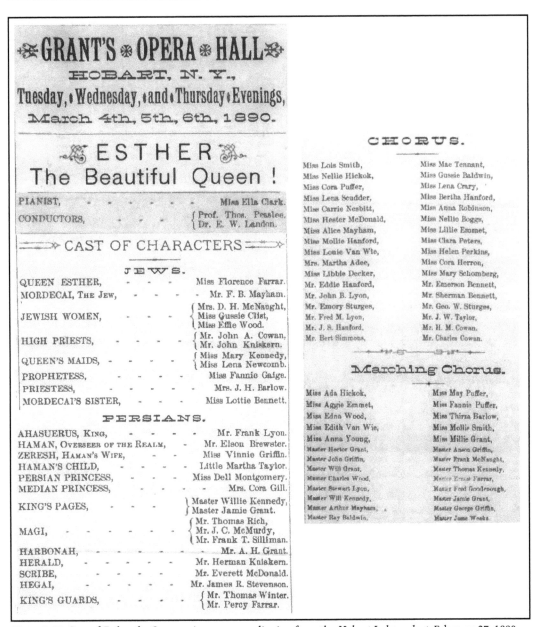

Figure 2-12. Cast of *Esther the Queen*—A newspaper clipping from the *Hobart Independent,* February 27, 1890.

Figure 2-13. Grant's Opera House circa 2018. (© Lori T. Andersen. Reprinted with permission.)

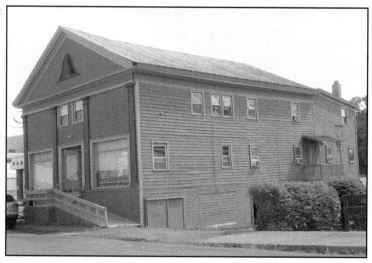

Figure 2-14. Old postcard of Grant's Opera House in the foreground on the left side and the St. Andrew's Masonic Lodge, No. 289 in the foreground on the right side. (Reprinted with permission from the Hobart Historical Society, Hobart, New York.)

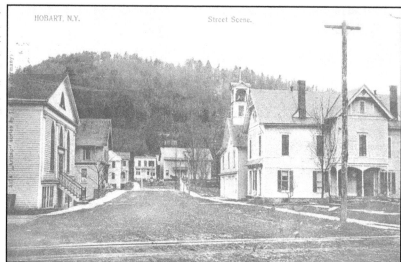

Figure 2-15a and Figure 2-15b. Hobart Historical Society circa 2018 and a photograph of the plaque indicating it was the previous home of St. Andrew's Masonic Lodge, No. 289, F. & A. M. and has been placed on the National Register of Historic Places. (© Lori T. Andersen. Reprinted with permission.)

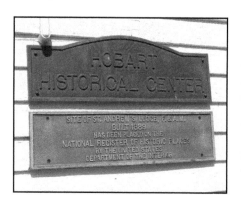

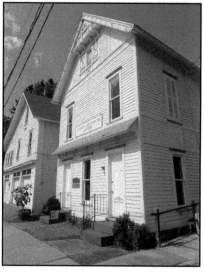

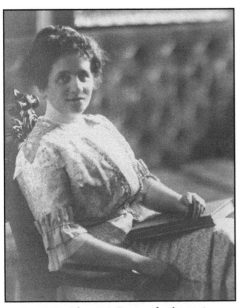

Figure 2-16. Eleanor. Date of photo is unknown. (Reprinted with permission from the Research Library at the Fenimore Art Museum, Cooperstown, New York, John Davenport Clarke Papers, Coll. No. 12, Box 9, MWC.)

February 1890. The fair was held in the hall of St. Andrew's Lodge, No. 289, the building that now houses the Hobart Historical Society ("The Masonic Fair", 1890) (Figures 2-15a and 2-15b). Eleanor maintained a connection with St. Peter's Episcopal Church, and in August 1906 she traveled back to Hobart from her residence in Chicago to help with the St. Peter's Church Ladies' Guild Bazaar. Eleanor was in charge of decorating the Grant's Opera House for this fundraising event ("Ladies Guild Bazaar", 1906) (Figure 2-16).

NURSING TRAINING

In May 1892, her father announced that Eleanor had accepted a position as a junior matron at the Elmira Hospital in Elmira, New York to continue her studies in medicine and that she would be paid well for her work ("Miss Ella, Daughter of Ex-sheriff Clark...", 1892; "The Ward Inquest Closed", 1892). While the author did not find any information about her prior interest or studies in medicine, Eleanor Clarke did go to Elmira to work in nursing and is listed in the 1893 Elmira city business directory as a "nurse AOMH" (Arnot Ogden Memorial Hospital) (Williams, 1892, p. 136). Arnot Ogden Hospital Training School in Elmira, New York was established in July 1889. They offered a two-year training program for nurses, and like other nurse training programs at that time, they provided a stipend (Hare & Kieffer, 2012, p. 65; United States, 1896, p. 2195). While a 1923 news article states she was a trained nurse, ("Illustrated Lecture", 1923), no record of her completing any type of formal nursing training was found by the author. Eleanor left Arnot Ogden Memorial Hospital sometime in 1893, possibly to pursue a relationship with Robert E. Slagle, whom she married in April 1894.

GETTING MARRIED

The Courtship

Little is known about Eleanor's activities during the second half of 1893 through April 1894 when she married Robert E. Slagle. News articles from that time began to describe her travels to various cities and states and then her subsequent marriage in April 1894. In July 1893, Eleanor, still a resident of Elmira, visited her Aunt Frances in Hobart and then traveled to Albany, New York ("Hobart", 1893). In September of that year, Eleanor and her Aunt Frances traveled to visit a friend, Mrs. B. F. Lee (Mary) of Rockford, Illinois, a city outside of Chicago. Eleanor and Aunt Frances then visited Chicago, most likely to see the 1893

World's Columbian Exposition in Chicago. After their visit to Chicago, Aunt Frances returned to Hobart and Eleanor traveled to Kansas. Eleanor stopped to visit with Mrs. Lee again on her return trip from Kansas before returning home to New York ("Purely Personal", 1893a, 1893b) (Figure 2-17). No further information about her life activities was found until the announcement of her upcoming wedding to Robert E. Slagle on April 19, 1894 ("Coming Wedding at Hobart", 1894). While initially pursuing a career in nursing at a time when there were few women in the workforce and opportunities were generally limited to teachers, nurses, or seamstresses, she opted for marriage as many women did.

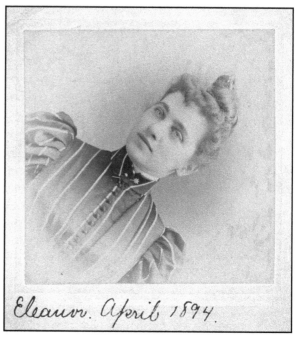

Figure 2-17. Eleanor in April 1894, the month she was married to Robert E. Slagle. (Reprinted with permission of the Research Library at the Fenimore Art Museum, Cooperstown, New York, John Davenport Clarke Papers, Coll. No. 12, Box 9, MWC.)

Eleanor's fiancée, Robert Ellsworth Slagle, was born in Exeter, Illinois in October 1863 to Reverend Peter Slagle of the Methodist Episcopal Church and Cordelia (Bean) Slagle. Robert had an older brother, Edward Rollin Slagle, and two younger sisters, Nellie Florence Slagle (Harnly) and Anna Daisy Slagle (McBratney). Two other sisters died in childhood (Madden, 1901, p. 122; U. S. Census Bureau, 1900). When he married Eleanor, Robert was an employee of the Pullman Palace Car Company. He started working for Pullman Palace Car Company in the late 1880s and continued to work for the company in various positions for approximately 30 years (Hoye's Kansas City Directory, 1905, p. 1046; The Lakeside Annual Directory of the City of Chicago, 1887, p. 1440; The Railroad Gazette, 1906, p. 171).

Since Eleanor was from New York and Robert was from Chicago, mystery surrounds the occasions of their meeting and courtship. Where and when did Eleanor Clark meet Robert E. Slagle, her future husband? Since Robert worked for the Pullman Palace Car Company, did she meet him while she was traveling by train? Was her July 1893 trip to Albany an occasion to tell her friend Lavina Griffin, a resident of Albany, of her engagement and ask her to be a bridesmaid? Did she go to Chicago in October 1893 chaperoned by Aunt Frances to be courted by Robert? Did Mrs. B. F. Lee of Rockford, Illinois, one of their wedding guests in April 1894, act as the hostess for their possible courting in October 1893? While we may never know the details of where they met and how they fell in love, their wedding was described in detail in a number of newspapers, the custom of the time.

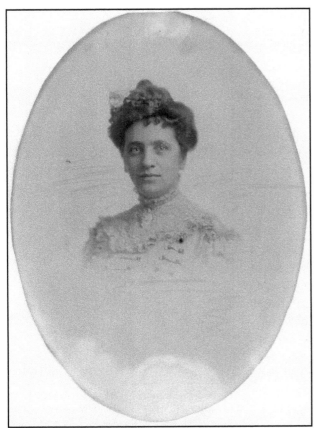

Figure 2-18. Eleanor circa April 1894, possibly a photo of Eleanor in her wedding dress. (Reprinted with permission from the Research Library at the Fenimore Art Museum, Cooperstown, New York, John Davenport Clarke Papers, Coll. No. 12, Box 7.)

The Wedding

Miss Eleanor Mai [sic] Clarke, the daughter of ex-sheriff William J. Clark, was married to Mr. Robert E. Slagle of Chicago on Thursday, April 19, 1894 at noon. The Rev. Thomas Burrows was the officiating rector of the ceremony that took place at St. Peter's Episcopal Church in Hobart, New York. Miss Gage was the organist for the wedding ceremony. Mr. R. Boyd of Chicago was best man for his friend Robert Slagle. Ushers included Messrs. F. D. Merritt, Crabtree, and Chester, all of Chicago; Mr. John D. Clarke the brother of the bride; Hon. James. R. Cowan, of Hobart; and J. Gould Barlow of Grand Gorge. Miss Mary C. Hanford of Hobart served as a bridesmaid and Miss Lavina E. Griffin of Albany served as the maid of honor ("A Fashionable Wedding", 1894; "Miss Clarke Wedded to R. C. Slagle" [sic], 1894). Miss Hanford was dressed in "white silk and Egyptian lace, with bouquet of pink roses" and Miss Griffin "in a gown of pink and white taffeta over a skirt of white lace and pink silk, and with pink crepe yoke and sleeves. She wore a large hat of Neapolitan, trimmed with pink roses and velvet, and Cusin roses" ("Of Interest to Albanians", 1894) (Figure 2-18).

> The bride's gown was of the most becoming silver gray crepon over a skirt of gray and white striped moire brocade, with flouncings of Duchesse lace and with shoes and gloves of gray suede. She wore a large Gainsborough hat of straw, trimmed with gray plumes, pink moire and roses. ("Of Interest to Albanians", 1894)

Miss Frances Clarke, the bride's aunt, gave a breakfast at the Clark family homestead after the ceremony. Among the guests were Miss Isabelle Kirchner, Mrs. J. Webster Griffin, Mr. Frank Gilbert, Mr. G. E. Graham of Albany, Mrs. M. W. Lee of Rockford, Illinois, and Mr. Edward Slagle—brother of the groom and assistant general manager of the Pullman Palace Car Company in Chicago, Illinois. An Albany, New York newspaper reported that Mr. and Mrs. Slagle will be "at home" after May, at "The Amazon," Forty-second street, Chicago ("Of Interest to Albanians", 1894).

The newly married couple's arrival in Chicago coincided with the Pullman Strike that started in May 1894 in Chicago. The Panic of 1893, an economic depression, prompted the

Pullman Palace Car Company to decrease the wages of its factory employees. In turn, the Pullman employees went on strike and the American Railroad Union started a boycott, paralyzing railroad travel. The ensuing riots and violence prompted President Grover Cleveland to take steps, including sending in the United States Army, to end the conflict. No information was found regarding any personal effect the strike may have had on the Slagles.

Married Life

Information gleaned from archival newspaper articles, census records, and city directories indicate that the couple lived in Chicago from 1894 to 1896, from 1898 to 1903, and again from 1907 to 1910. In between these times they lived in St. Louis from 1896 to 1897, and in Kansas City, Missouri from 1904 to 1907 (all dates are approximate). Robert's job involved travel and frequent absences from home. On several occasions during their early years of marriage, Mrs. Slagle returned to New York for extended stays to visit with friends and family. She also traveled to other parts of the country (Figure 2-19). She enjoyed spending time in the Thousand Islands

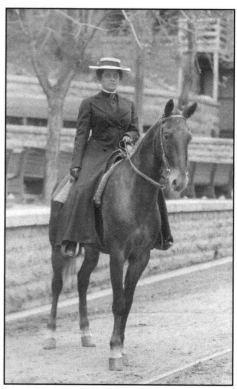

Figure 2-19. Eleanor on horseback, circa late 1890s to early 1900s. (Reprinted with permission of the Research Library at the Fenimore Art Museum, Cooperstown, New York, John Davenport Clarke Papers, Coll. No. 12, Box 9, MWC.)

with friends and family ("Glenfield", 1908, 1910b, 1912, 1915b). The Thousand Islands, an archipelago of islands located in the St. Lawrence River between the northern border of New York and southern border of Canada, offered a peaceful retreat for Mrs. Slagle and her friends. In October 1907, Mrs. Slagle traveled to Atlantic City, New Jersey, another popular tourist destination, sending a photo postcard home to Mr. William Happ, her mother's second husband (Figures 2-20a and 2-20b). On most occasions, her husband Robert, or Rob as she called him, did not accompany her ("About the Folks", 1897, 1898a, 1898b, 1898c, 1905; "Society's Busy Whirl", 1901; "Those Who Come and Go", 1907; "What Society is Doing", 1902). In March 1910, after 16 years of marriage, Rob and Eleanor separated (Slagle vs Slagle, 1914). They had no children. Although the reason for the failure of their marriage is not known, Rob's frequent job related absences from home may have strained the marriage.

FAMILY TIES

Eleanor had close relationships with many in her extended family, but was particularly close with her father, her brother, and her Aunt Frances. After her parent's divorce, Eleanor had minimal contact with her mother, Emma, until the death of her father in 1897. At that time, Eleanor and her mother reconnected and maintained a close relationship until Emma's death in 1920.

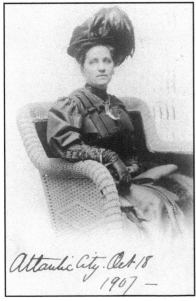

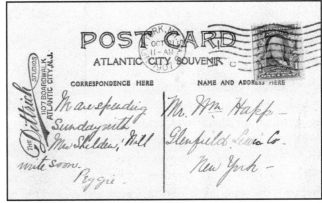

Figure 2-20. (A) Eleanor Clarke Slagle pictured on a photo postcard from Atlantic City. Photo postcards were introduced in 1907 and allowed tourists to send home a message to friends and family about their travels. (Reprinted with permission from the Research Library at the Fenimore Art Museum, Cooperstown, New York, John Davenport Clarke Papers, Coll. No. 12, Box 9, MWC.) (B) The government first allowed a "split back" postcard in 1907, allowing space for a written message along with the recipient's address. Note that Eleanor signed her message "Peggie". Her family often called her Peggie or Aunt Peggie. (Reprinted with permission from the Research Library at the Fenimore Art Museum, Cooperstown, New York, John Davenport Clarke Papers, Coll. No. 12, Box 9, MWC.)

Relationship With her Father

Eleanor remained close to her father after her parent's separation, traveling with him to DeLand, Florida in 1892 for an extended winter vacation and accompanying him to local social events on occasion. This close relationship continued during the early years of her marriage as well ("Local and Miscellaneous", 1891; "The Ward Inquest Closed", 1892; "Wedding Bells", 1887) so it was not surprising that at the end of 1896, when he was in poor health, William J. Clarke traveled to St. Louis to live his last days at the home of his daughter ("Local and Miscellaneous", 1896). On January 30, 1897, he died at her home at 3819 Olive Street in St. Louis (Missouri Death Records [Microfilm], 1850-1931). His body was returned to Hobart, New York where a funeral service was held at the Clark family homestead. The service was attended by members of the Grand Army of the Republic (G. A. R.) from Hobart and many of the Masons from St. Andrew's Lodge in Hobart. He was buried in Locust Hill Cemetery ("Ex-Sheriff Clark Dead", 1897).

In June 1929, long after her father's death, Eleanor Clarke Slagle sent a prayer book that belonged to the Strawberry Chapel in South Carolina and a letter to Bishop Albert S. Thomas of the diocese of South Carolina. The letter explained that Mrs. Slagle found the prayer book in her father's effects after his death and that she wanted to return the prayer book to the rightful owner. The inscription, written in pencil on the flyleaf in the prayer book, read:

> This book belongs to Strawberry Chapple, South Carolina. It was taken from the church of this parish by a Rebbie Soldier, carried some distance, thrown away, and picked up by me in May, 1865. (Signed), Wm. J. Clarke, Lieut., 144th N. Y. V. ("Bishop Receives", 1929, p. 12; "Plan Service at Historic Church", 1929, p. 2)

Bond With her Aunt Frances and her Brother John

Eleanor and her brother John maintained strong ties to each other throughout their lives and they both maintained strong ties with their Aunt Frances, who was always there to help. Aunt Frances, who became the matriarch of the Clark family and owner of the Clark family homestead in Hobart, provided a safe, welcoming environment for the family. The homestead was the location of a number of the Clark family's births, parties, weddings, deaths, and funerals. Eleanor and John spent numerous school vacations there and when Eleanor became seriously ill in the summer of 1889, she stayed with Aunt Frances who cared for her until she recovered. Even when Eleanor and John each lived out of state or out of town, they continued to visit Aunt Frances until her death in 1906 ("Home and Vicinity", 1886, 1888a, 1889; "Personals", 1887, 1889b; "Hobart Happenings", 1902, 1903, 1904).

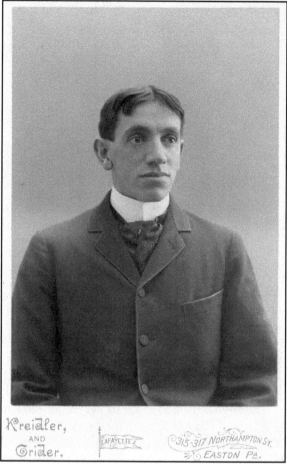

Figure 2-21. John Davenport Clarke circa 1898. (Reprinted with permission from the Research Library at the Fenimore Art Museum, Cooperstown, New York, John Davenport Clarke Papers, Coll. No. 12, Box 7.)

In contrast to Eleanor's sketchy educational record, her brother John's educational record is more complete. John attended the Delaware Academy, graduating in 1886 from the academic program (Delaware Academy, 1890). He attended the Delaware Literary Institute in Franklin, New York for a short time in 1891 (Colcord, 1892) and then Philips Andover Academy, a preparatory school in Andover, Massachusetts in 1892 (Phillips Exeter Academy, 1892). John returned to Delaware Academy to complete the preparatory program there, graduating in 1894. He continued his studies at Lafayette College in Easton, Pennsylvania, graduating in June 1898 ("About the Folks", 1898a), and then enrolled in the Princeton Theological Seminary in New Jersey in September 1898 with the intent to enter the ministry ("About the Folks", 1898b) (Figure 2-21). After a few months, he left the seminary program and went out west for health reasons, most likely suffering from tuberculosis (Stone, 1898). John then completed post-graduate courses at Colorado College in Colorado Springs in June 1899 (Slocum, 1905; United States, 1934, p. 5), and in the fall of that year, John was hired by Colorado College to teach rhetoric and elocution. He was also named superintendent of the athletic department at Colorado College ("In Village and Town", 1899; "Local and

Miscellaneous", 1899). It was there that he met his future wife Marian Kingsley Williams ("Mrs. Clarke...", 1927).

John and Marian were married on June 6, 1905 in her parent's home in Wyoming. After the wedding, the couple made their home in Rockledge on the Hudson in New York ("Clarke-Williams", 1905; "Weddings Past and to Come", 1905). John, who by that time was working for United States Steel, moved to Duluth, Minnesota with his new wife when he was promoted to assistant to the president of the company ("John D. Clark... ", 1905). It was in Duluth that John Duncan Clarke, John and Marian's son and Eleanor's nephew, was born on September 16, 1906. At the age of six John Duncan, nicknamed Jack, contracted infantile paralysis that affected his ability to use his right arm for the rest of his life (Clarke, 1928). The Clarke family eventually moved back to New York where the elder John decided to continue his education, earning his law degree from Brooklyn Law School in 1911 (United States, 1934, p. 5).

FINDING A CAREER PATH

In the latter part of the first decade of the 1900s, at the same time that her brother was changing his career path, Mrs. Slagle started to take an interest in social and political issues. Finding a new purpose in life, she became a member of the Woman's City Club of Chicago ("New Members, ...", 1918) and a member of the Political Equality League in Chicago during the Illinois suffrage movement (Chicago American, 1939). In 1910, she gave a presentation to the a Women's Review Club in New York State on the topic of political democracy, a system in which all people share political power and participate in politics directly or indirectly through their elected representatives ("Glenfield", 1910a; Slagle, n.d.). Mrs. Slagle's presentation was given at a time when women were seeking the right participate in the political process—the right to vote through the women's suffrage movement. With Mrs. Slagle's newfound interests and her brother John's new career, both were headed for careers in public service just like their father years before.

REFERENCES

A fashionable wedding. (1894, April 25). *Delaware Gazette,* p. 3. Retrieved from http://nyshistoricnewspapers. org/lccn/sn83030838/1894-04-25/ed-1/seq-3/

About the folks. (1897, February 27). *Stamford Recorder/Hobart Recorder,* p. 1. Retrieved from www.fultonhistory. com

About the folks. (1898a, June 25). *Stamford Recorder/Hobart Recorder,* p. unknown. Retrieved from www.fulton-history.com

About the folks. (1898b, September 3). *Stamford Recorder/Hobart Recorder,* p. unknown. Retrieved from www. fultonhistory.com

About the folks. (1898c, October 22). *Stamford Recorder/Hobart Recorder,* p. 1. Retrieved from www.fultonhistory.com

About the folks. (1905, September 16). *Hobart Independent,* p. 1. Retrieved from www.fultonhistory.com

Being pushed along. (1895, May 18). *Watertown Herald,* p. 5. Retrieved from http://nyshistoricnewspapers.org/lccn/sn85054447/1895-05-18/ed-1/seq-5/

Bishop receives old prayer book—Volume taken North by Union Soldier is restored to Strawberry Chapel. (1929, June 9). *Charleston News and Courier,* p. 12. Retrieved from www.genealogybank.com

Carthage. (1888, November 10). *Watertown Herald,* p. 1. Retrieved from http://nyshistoricnewspapers.org/lccn/sn85054447/1888-11-10/ed-1/seq-3/

Carthage. (1891, February 28). *Watertown Herald,* p. 2. Retrieved from http://nyshistoricnewspapers.org/lccn/sn85054447/1891-02-28/ed-1/seq-2/

Chicago American. (1939, July). Eleanor Clarke Slagle, occupational therapy founder, 'back home' for convention. *Chicago American,* no page number. Clipped newspaper article retrieved Archive of the American Occupational Therapy Association, Bethesda, MD.

Chicago School of Civics and Philanthropy. (1911). *Transcript: Slagle Eleanor Clarke.* University of Illinois-Chicago: CSCP Archives Collection.

Clark, E. J. vs. Clark, W. J. (1890). *Divorce papers, Case No. 394, August term, 1890.* Records of the Surrogate's Court, County of Susquehanna, Montrose, Pennsylvania.

Clark, E. J. vs. Clark, W. J. (1891). *Report of Master.* Susquehanna County, PA; Court Case #394 August term, 1890 (Divorce).

Clarke-Williams. (1905, June 22). *Denver Rocky Mountain News,* p. 7. Retrieved from www.genealogybank.com

Clarke, J. D. (1928, June 30). *Letter to E. Lyman.* Research Library at the Fenimore Art Museum, (Collection 12, Box 35, Folder 19), Cooperstown, NY.

Clarke, J. D. (1931, June 29). *Letter to E. C. Slagle.* Research Library at the Fenimore Art Museum, (Collection 12, Box 4, Folder 6), Cooperstown, NY.

Colcord, E. J. (1892). *Reference letter from E. J. Colcord for John D. Clarke on January 28, 1892.* Research Library at the Fenimore Art Museum, (Collection 12, Box 5, Folder 1), Cooperstown, NY.

Coming wedding at Hobart. (1894, April 4). *Delaware Gazette,* p. 3. Retrieved from http://nyshistoricnewspapers.org/lccn/sn83030838/1894-04-04/ed-1/seq-3/

Delaware Academy. (1890). Catalogue and circular of Delaware Academy for the five years from 1885 to 1890: Sixty-seventh to seventy-first year, inclusive. *Delaware Express Print.* (Available at the H. Fletcher Davidson Library Archives, Delaware County Historical Association. Delhi, New York).

Delaware Academy Central School District at Delhi. (2021). *About Delaware Academy.* Retrieved from http://delawareacs.ss10.sharpschool.com/our_district/about_delaware_academy

Delaware County Clerk. (1869, February 24). *[Deed to William J. Clark, grantee, from Maria Hanford (deceased), grantor (Ebenezer Gallup, executor for deceased)]* Liber 69, pages 65-66. Records of the County Clerk, County of Delaware, Delhi, New York. Available at Delaware County Courthouse, Delhi, New York.

Ella Clark and Jennie Middlemist… (1885, June 17). *Delaware Gazette,* p. 3. Retrieved from http://nyshistoricnewspapers.org/lccn/sn83030838/1885-06-17/ed-1/seq-3/

Ex-Sheriff Clark dead. (1897, February 6). *Stamford Recorder,* p. 1. Retrieved from www.fultonhistory.com

Ex-Sheriff Clark has gone to spend…. (1886, October 20). *Delaware Gazette,* p. 3. http://nyshistoricnewspapers.org/lccn/sn83030838/1886-10-20/ed-1/seq-3/

G.A.R. England Post No. 142. (1885, January 19). *G.A.R. Book of minutes,* No. 2, England Post No. 142. H. Fletcher Davidson Library Archives, Delaware County Historical Association. Delhi, New York.

Glenfield. (1908, July 16). *Journal and Republican,* p. 8. Retrieved from http://nyshistoricnewspapers.org/lccn/sn83031789/1908-07-16/ed-1/seq-8/

Glenfield. (1910a, January 13). *Journal and Republican and Lowville Times,* p. unknown. Retrieved from www.fultonhistory.com

Glenfield. (1910b, July 21). *Journal and Republican and Lowville Times,* p. 2. Retrieved from www.fultonhistory.comGlenfield. (1912, September 6). Watertown Daily Times, p. 9. Retrieved from www.genealogybank.com

Glenfield. (1915a, April 29). *Journal and Republican and Lowville Times,* p. 2. Retrieved from http://nyshistoricnewspapers.org/lccn/sn93063681/1915-04-29/ed-1/seq-2/

Glenfield. (1915b, August 5). *Journal and Republican and Lowville Times,* p. 2. Retrieved from http://nyshistoricnewspapers.org/lccn/sn93063681/1915-08-05/ed-1/seq-2/

Grant's Opera Hall. (1890, February 27). *Hobart Independent,* p. 2. Retrieved from www.fultonhistory.com

Happenings of particular interest to Stamford. (1927, April 6). *Stamford Mirror-Recorder,* p. 5. Retrieved from www.fultonhistory.com

Hare, J. E., & Kieffer, J. A. (2012). The Arnot Ogden Memorial Hospital and St. Joseph's Hospital (pp. 61-74). In *Elmira.* Arcadia Publishing.

Hobart. (1893, July 11). *Stamford Mirror,* p. 3. Retrieved from www.fultonhistory.com

Hobart happenings. (1902, July 26). *Stamford Recorder.* Retrieved from www.fultonhistory.com

Hobart happenings. (1903, March 21). *Stamford Recorder.* Retrieved from www.fultonhistory.com

Hobart happenings. (1904, January 4). *Stamford Recorder,* p. 1. Retrieved from www.fultonhistory.com

Home and vicinity. (1886, July 22). *Hobart Independent,* p. 3. Retrieved from www.fultonhistory.com

Home and vicinity. (1888a, August 23). Pleasant party. *Hobart Independent,* p. 3. Retrieved from www.fultonhistory.com

Home and vicinity. (1888b, November 15). *Hobart Independent,* p. 3. Retrieved from www.fultonhistory.com

Home and vicinity. (1889, July 11). *Hobart Independent,* p. 3. Retrieved from www.fultonhistory.com

Hoye's Kansas City Directory. (1905). *Hoye Directory Company.* Retrieved from www.ancestry.com

Illustrated lecture. (1923, February 15). *Gowanda Enterprise,* p. 1. Retrieved from www.fultonhistory.com

In village and town. (1899, September 2). *Hobart Independent.* Retrieved from www.fultonhistory.com

John D. Clarke… (1905, December 13). *Carthage Republican,* p. 5. Retrieved from www.fultonhistory.com

Ladies Guild Bazaar. (1906, August 11). *Hobart Independent,* p. 1. Retrieved from www.fultonhistory.com

Local and miscellaneous. (1891, February 18). *Delaware Gazette,* p. 3. Retrieved from http://nyshistoricnewspapers.org/lccn/sn83030838/1891-02-18/ed-1/seq-3/

Local and miscellaneous. (1896, December 30). *Delaware Gazette,* p. 3. Retrieved from http://nyshistoricnewspapers.org/lccn/sn83030838/1896-12-30/ed-1/seq-3/

Local and miscellaneous. (1899, September 13). *Delaware Gazette,* p. 3. Retrieved from http://nyshistoricnewspapers.org/lccn/sn83030838/1899-09-13/ed-1/seq-3/

Madden, F. B. (Ed.). (1901). Rev. Peter Slagle. In *Journal and records of the seventy-eighth session Illinois Annual Conference of the Methodist Episcopal Church,* pp. 122-123. Illinois State Register.

Meagley, J. G. (2014). *A look back at Hobart, NY on the 125th Anniversary of the Village Incorporation, 1888-2013.* Hobart Historical Society.

Milo Deyo Dies; Concert Pianist. (1925, February 20). *Brooklyn Daily Eagle,* p. 17. Retrieved from www.newspapers.com

Miss Clarke wedded to R. C. Slagle. (1894, April 20). *Chicago Daily Tribune,* p. 2. Retrieved from www.newspapers.com

Miss Ella, daughter of Ex-sheriff Clark… (1892, May 25). *Delaware Gazette,* p. 3. Retrieved from http://nyshistoricnewspapers.org/lccn/sn83030838/1892-05-25/ed-1/seq-3/

Miss Ella May Clark... (1886, June 23). *Delaware Gazette,* p. 3. Retrieved from http://nyshistoricnewspapers.org/lccn/sn83030838/1886-06-23/ed-1/seq-3/

Miss Fannie Bordon, Miss Ella Clark… (1886, September 1). *Delaware Gazette,* p. 3. Retrieved from http://nyshistoricnewspapers.org/lccn/sn83030838/1886-09-01/ed-1/seq-3/

Miss Gussie Bowne…. (1887, May 4). *Delaware Gazette,* p. 3. Retrieved from http://nyshistoricnewspapers.org/lccn/sn83030838/1887-05-04/ed-1/seq-3/

Missouri Death Records [Microfilm]. (1850-1931). *City of St. Louis, Health Department, certificate of death for Wm. J. Clark-1897.* Missouri State Archives; Jefferson City, MO. Retrieved from www.ancestry.com

Mrs. Clarke is heartily welcomed back to Capital's social life. (1927, January 28). *Binghamton Press,* p. 19. Retrieved from www.newspapers.com

New Members, September 25 to November 21, 1918. (1918, December). *Woman's City Club Bulletin,* 7(8), p. 20-21.

New York, State Census. (1875). *Town of Stamford, County of Delaware. Line 11 – 14, June 9, 1875, p. 10. FHL microfilm 832,851.* Retrieved from http://familysearch.com

Of interest to Albanians. (1894, April 20). *Albany Morning Express,* p. 5. Retrieved from www.fultonhistory.com

Pennsylvania, County Marriages, 1885-1950 [database on-line]. (2016, December). *Marriage certificate of Wm. A. Happ and Emma J. Clark, February 25, 1891.* Retrieved from www.familysearch.com.

Personals. (1887, August 24). *Delaware Gazette,* p. 3. Retrieved from http://nyshistoricnewspapers.org/lccn/sn83030838/1887-08-24/ed-1/seq-3/

Personals. (1889a, May 9). *Hobart Independent,* p. 3. Retrieved from www.fultonhistory.comPersonals. (1889b, June 20). Hobart Independent, p. 3. Retrieved from www.fultonhistory.com

Purely personal. (1893a, September 20). *Morning Star,* p. 8. Retrieved from www.genealogybank.com

Purely personal. (1893b, November 3). *Morning Star,* p. 8. Retrieved from www.genealogybank.com

Phillips Exeter Academy. (1892). *Annual athletic meeting of Phillips Exeter Academy vs. Phillips Andover Academy held on Exeter Campus June 4, 1892.* Phillips Exeter. (Available at the Research Library at the Fenimore Art Museum).

Plan service at historic church. (1929, December 14). *Charleston News and Courier,* p. 12. Retrieved from www.genealogybank.com

Reward will be presented… (1885, January 7). *Delaware Gazette,* p. 5. Retrieved from http://nyshistoricnewspapers.org/lccn/sn83030838/1885-01-07/ed-1/seq-5/

R.V. LeRay Co. (1889). *LeRay's Poughkeepsie city directory for the year ending May 1, 1889.* R.V. LeRay. Retrieved from www.ancestry.com

Slagle, E. C. (n.d.). *Experience of Eleanor Clarke Slagle.* Archives of the American Occupational Therapy Association.

Slagle, E. C. vs Slagle, R. E. (1914, July 3). *Decree for divorce.* Circuit Court of Cook County, B 115.

Slocum, W. F. (1905, May 3). *Reference letter re: John D. Clarke.* Research Library at the Fenimore Art Museum, (Collection 12, Box 5, Folder 1), Cooperstown, NY.

St. Peter's Episcopal Church (Hobart, NY), Vosburgh, R. W., & New York Genealogical and Biographical Society. (1921). *Records of St. Peter's Episcopal Church in the village of Hobart, town of Stamford, Delaware County, NY.* (Supplement, August 1921). New York City: publisher not identified.

Society's busy whirl. (1901, September 7). *Hobart Independent,* no page number. Retrieved from www.fultonhistory.com

Stone, W. A. (1898). *Reference letter from W. A. Stone for John D. Clarke on December 2, 1898.* Research Library at the Fenimore Art Museum, (Collection 12, Box 5, Folder 1), Cooperstown, NY.

Susquehanna County, Commonwealth of Pennsylvania. (1891). *Certificate of marriage—W. A. Happ & Emma J. Clark.* Author. Retrieved from Pennsylvania, County Marriages, 1885-1950, (https://familysearch.org/ark:/61903/1:1:VF4D-JJH:24 June 2016). Retrieved from www.familysearch.org

The Lakeside Annual Directory of the City of Chicago. (1887). *The Chicago Directory Company.* Retrieved from www.ancestry.com

The Masonic Fair. (1890, February 13). *Hobart Independent,* p. 3. Retrieved from www.fultonhistory.com

The Railroad Gazette. (1906, December 21). Manufacturing and business. *Railroad Gazette: A Journal of Transportation, Engineering and Railroad News, 41,* 171. [In General News Section].

The Ward inquest closed. (1892, May 18). *Middletown Daily Times,* p. 7. Retrieved from www.newspapers.com

Those who come and go. (1907, August 3). *Hobart Independent,* p. 1. Retrieved from www.fultonhistory.com

Town tattle. (1905, March 29). *Carthage Republican,* p. 5. Retrieved from www.fultonhistory.com

Uncle Rube. (1889, January 10). *Hobart Independent,* p. unknown. Retrieved from www.fultonhistory.com

United States. (1896). *Report of the Commissioner of Education for the Year 1894-95, Volume 2: Table 7. Statistics of schools for training nurses, for 1894-1895* (pp. 2193-2195). United States Government Printing Office.

United States. (1934). *Memorial services held in the House of Representatives of the United States, together with remarks presented in eulogy of John D. Clarke: Late a representative from New York.* United States Government Printing Office.

U. S. Census Bureau. (1900). *Hyde Park Township, Supervisor's District No. 1, Cook County, Illinois, Chicago City, enumeration district (ED) 1086, Sheet 11, Line 35 – 36, June 6, 1900.* Microfilm: Retrieved from http://familysearch.com

Wedding bells. (1887, September 8). *Hobart Independent,* p. 3. Retrieved from www.fultonhistory.com

Weddings past and to come. (1905, June 17). *Hobart Independent,* p. 1. Retrieved from www.fultonhistory.com

Welch, E. L. (1897). *Historical souvenir of Delhi, NY.* Albany, NY.

What society is doing. (1902, August). *Hobart Independent.* Retrieved from www.fultonhistory.com

Williams, J. E. (1892). *Williams' directory of Elmira city and business directory of Horseheads.* Gazette Company, Book and Job Printers.

A New Purpose in Life for Eleanor Clarke Slagle

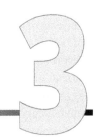

"The future belongs to those who believe in the beauty of their dreams."
Eleanor Roosevelt

Robert and Eleanor were living in Chicago in March 1910 when Robert left Eleanor and moved to Idaho to live with his sister, Mrs. Anna McBratney. While there were reports that their marriage was not a happy one, it is not known if there was a specific incident that precipitated this permanent separation. In January 1914, four years after the separation, Eleanor filed for divorce on the grounds of willful desertion. The divorce was granted on July 3, 1914 (Slagle vs. Slagle, 1914; U.S. Census Bureau, 1910).

Robert remained in Idaho working as a ticket agent for the railroad. In 1915, he married Gertrude Carter (1884–1986) ("Gertrude Slagle", 1986). They had one child, a daughter Roberta born in 1917 (U.S. Census Bureau, 1920). Robert died of a heart attack in September 1933 while visiting another sister, Mrs. Nellie Harnly, in Chicago ("Former Ticket Agent at Nampa Succumbs", 1933). His body was returned to Nampa, Idaho, where he is buried. In 1937, Eleanor described herself as a "long time widow" (Quiroga, 1995, p. 43-44), perhaps to avoid the questions and stigma associated with being divorced.

During the difficult time when her marriage failed and finally ended, Mrs. Slagle started to pursue her interest in the plight of those with mental and physical disabilities. Her resume states that:

> Covering a period of years of interest in the unfair social attitude toward the dependency of mentally and physically handicapped, followed by lectures on Social Economics by Professor Henderson, Chicago University, Jane Adams [sic], Hull House, Julia Lathrop, now of the Children's Bureau, I took up: ... Special course in occupations and educational methods, Chicago School of Civics and Philanthropy, now part of the University of Chicago, followed by a six months study of hospitals, charitable institutions, and dependency of mental and physical cases. (Slagle, n. d.).

Mrs. Slagle's New Professional Life

Mrs. Slagle was experiencing changes in her personal life at the same time the United States was experiencing a wave of activism with significant social and political reforms. As her resume states, Mrs. Slagle connected with women activists such as Jane Addams and Julia Lathrop of Hull House. She also became involved in women's organizations that promoted social and political reform—the Chicago Woman's Club, the Chicago Political Equality League, and the General Federation of Women's Clubs. Eleanor also started taking classes at the Chicago School of Civics and Philanthropy (CSCP). Formally established in 1908, the CSCP evolved as part of the settlement house movement's focus on humanitarian work and research. It was through her connection with Jane Addams and Julia Lathrop that Mrs. Slagle became interested in the new profession of occupational therapy.

Graham Taylor founded the Chicago Commons, a settlement house in Chicago that was modeled after Hull House. He began providing social work lectures, but wanted to expand the specialized educational programs in order to develop skilled humanitarian workers and researchers. To expand these educational programs, Taylor joined with other agencies to establish the CSCP to provide full training programs. In alignment with the Progressive Movement, the new school's objective was to "to promote through instruction, training, investigation, and publication the efficiency of civic, philanthropic and social work, and the improvement of living and working conditions" (Chicago School of Civics and Philanthropy, 1909, p. 9). Taylor was the first president and Julia Lathrop, from Hull House, was the first vice-president of the school. Jane Addams served as a member of the board of trustees (Chicago School of Civics and Philanthropy, 1909, p. 6). The CSCP eventually merged with the University of Chicago's Philanthropic Division in 1920 to become the University of Chicago School of Social Service Administration (University of Chicago Library, 2010).

In the summer of 1908, the CSCP offered a course to train attendants and nurses on the therapeutic use of occupation with patients with mental illness. Dr. Adolf Meyer, the renowned psychiatrist who was supportive of the use of occupation for treatment of patients with mental illness, had encouraged his personal friend and professional colleague Julia Lathrop to develop this course (Levine, 1987), a course that Mrs. Slagle took in 1911. By applying the concepts of moral treatment and the Arts and Crafts Movement, it was believed that engaging patients in occupations and getting them to use muscles and mind together in games, exercises, and handicrafts would re-educate and stimulate the patients and could provide a mental distraction from worrisome thoughts. Implementing these concepts and programs with patients with mental illness required training of the staff who were working with these patients. This was the type of training that the CSCP sought to provide for humanitarian workers. The CSCP also expected that, by improving the skills of nurses and attendants in institutions, it would increase their status and pay and, as a result, it would improve the ability of institutions to recruit qualified personnel (Chicago School of Civics and Philanthropy, 1911a, p. 14).

Mrs. Slagle started taking classes at the CSCP in 1910 (Slagle, n.d.). While she was taking courses in social economics, psychology, and recreation, a field work experience had a profound impact on Mrs. Slagle. Field work, or learning by doing, was an important part of the coursework at the CSCP. On a visit to the Kankakee State Hospital, Mrs. Slagle observed an unkempt woman secretly unraveling her undershirt. The woman was knitting a small child's shirt with the unraveled material, using two straightened hair pins as knitting needles.

Mrs. Slagle inquired if the shirt was for her little girl. The woman immediately brightened up, replied that she had four children, and then resumed her knitting. Through this experience, Mrs. Slagle realized the power of engagement in purposeful activity for these less fortunate people in state hospitals who, in most cases, lacked of meaningful activities. Because of that experience, she was determined to help those with mental illness (Illinois State Department of Public Welfare, 1939).

Encouraged by her mentor, Julia Lathrop, Mrs. Slagle enrolled in the special summer course in occupations, a five-week course that ran from June 26 to July 28, 1911. Lectures and practical activities focused on handicrafts and various forms of recreation, deemed to be the "two equally important parts" of occupation, as some might be stimulated by handicrafts and some by recreation (Chicago School of Civics and Philanthropy, 1911b, pp. 35-36). Handicraft lessons included learning leatherwork, metal work, bookbinding, braiding, working with clay, paper and cardboard work skills, as well as ways to adapt these crafts for those in institutions. Lessons in recreational activities included indoor and outdoor games, dancing, physical training, and play.

According to Mrs. Slagle's resume, after completing the occupations course she was hired as a consultant by Newberry State Hospital in Newberry, Michigan (previously known as Upper Peninsula Asylum for the Insane) for six months (Slagle, n.d.). Using the CSCP course as a model, she taught a course on occupations and amusements for employees and patients. When Mrs. Slagle completed her assignment to establish the occupations and amusements department, a graduate attendant was assigned to carry out the work (Newberry State Hospital, 1913, p. 24). After her assignment at Newberry State Hospital, Mrs. Slagle was hired by the State Hospital in Central Islip, New York (Long Island) for six months. There she organized the State Hospital's re-educational classes and established a schedule of activity for the patients (Slagle, n.d.; Slagle, 1936).

In July 1912, Mrs. Slagle returned to Chicago where the CSCP had arranged for her to co-teach the fifth summer session of the occupations course with Mr. Edward F. Worst. Mr. Worst was the superintendent of schools in Joliet, Illinois, and the charge teacher for the handicrafts part of previous courses at CSCP (Chicago School of Civics and Philanthropy, 1911a, p. 17; 1912, p. 39). In contrast to previous summer courses, arrangements were made to teach this fifth course "in a state hospital for the insane, where practical value of the work can be demonstrated by actual practice by attendants and nurses who are taking the training" (Chicago School of Civics and Philanthropy, 1912, March, p. 39) (Table 3-1).

In 1913, a new opportunity presented itself for Mrs. Slagle. She moved to Baltimore, Maryland to establish the occupational therapy department at the new Henry Phipps Psychiatric Clinic at Johns Hopkins Hospital. Henry Phipps was a wealthy philanthropist who was moved by Clifford Beers book *A Mind that Found Itself* and the subsequent Mental Hygiene Movement. He donated a large sum of money to cover the cost of constructing a building to house a psychiatric center at the Johns Hopkins Hospital in Baltimore, Maryland (Johns Hopkins Hospital, 1915, p. 4). The center, headed by the renowned psychiatrist Dr. Adolf Meyer, officially opened in mid-April 1913. As part of the coverage of the clinic's opening, an article in *The Evening Sun* (a Baltimore newspaper) reported that,

> Mrs. Slagle, of Chicago, who is now installing the occupational and entertaining system in the Kings Park State Hospital, New York, will join the clinic forces on May 1 to take charge of the entertainment of the patients, to amuse them and provide occupations and employment for them. ("World's Greatest Medical Men Here…", 1913)

TABLE 3-1. MRS. SLAGLE'S WORK HISTORY AND PROFESSIONAL POSITIONS

Year	Full-Time Work	Consultant Work	Other (Time Limited and Volunteer Positions)
1911		Upper Peninsula State Hospital, Newberry, Michigan (1911) and State Hospital, Central Islip, Long Island, New York (1911 to 1912)	
1912	Director of Occupational Therapy, Phipps Psychiatric Clinic, Baltimore (April 1912 to 1914; 1 year 9 months)		
1913		Started Community Workshop, Chicago—Illinois Society of Mental Hygiene (1913 to 1914)	Lectured for Chicago School of Civics and Philanthropy (1913 to 1914)
1914 to 1915	Director of Occupational Therapy for Community Workshop and training school for OTs (Henry B. Favill School of Occupations (1914 to 1917)		
1916		Organized occupational classroom at Bedford Reformatory, Social Hygiene Laboratory, Bedford Hills, NY	Performed survey for Montefiore Hospital and Country Sanitarium (1 week)
1917	General Superintendent of Occupational Therapy for Illinois Department of Public Welfare (1917 to 1920) Continued as Director of Community Workshop		Performed Survey for Military Hospitals Commission, Canada (2 weeks) *Volunteer:* Vice-president of NSPOT

(continued)

TABLE 3-1. MRS. SLAGLE'S WORK HISTORY AND PROFESSIONAL POSITIONS (CONTINUED)

Year	Full-Time Work	Consultant Work	Other (Time Limited and Volunteer Positions)
1918	Supervisor of Reconstruction Aides in Occupational Therapy (December 1918 to March 1919; resigned due to serious bout with influenza).	Supervised/taught occupational therapy classes for Chicago Chapter of the Red Cross Consultant to U.S. Public Health Service Consultant to NY State Hospital Commission Consultant to Military Hospital Commission, Canada Consultant to U.S. Surgeon General's Office	Consultant to St. Louis School of Occupational Therapy and Philadelphia School of Occupational Therapy *Volunteer:* Vice-president of NSPOT
1919			*Volunteer:* President of NSPOT (1919 to 1920)
1920	Executive Director of the Occupation Therapy Society of New York (June 1920 to October 1921; 1 year)	Consultant to U.S. Public Health Service	Consultant to National Tuberculosis Association
1921			*Volunteer:* Secretary-Treasurer of NSPOT/AOTA (1921 to 1937)
1922 to 1942	Director of Occupational Therapy for New York State Hospital Commission—later named Department of Mental Hygiene (July 1, 1922 to September 18, 1942)		

Note: Primary sources are Mrs. Slagle's resume, journal articles, and newspaper articles. While these sources are not always consistent in dates of service, possibly because of overlapping consultancy or part-time jobs, the table attempts to use best evidence in listing positions and dates.

As part of her work at the Henry Phipps Psychiatric Clinic, Mrs. Slagle instituted a program of habit training with chronically ill patients based on Dr. Adolf Meyer's belief that a person's disorganized habits contributed to chronic mental illness (Meyer, 1922/1977). Daily schedules were established for patients to follow to ensure healthy living habits and a balance of work, rest, and play. Each day at the same time patients would perform certain occupations such as bathing, dressing, eating meals, work activities, recreational activities, and sleep, with the goal that patients would eventually follow the daily routine independently (Peloquin, 1991).

While she was living in Baltimore, Mrs. Slagle met Dr. William Rush Dunton Jr., the psychiatrist in charge of the occupations and recreation program at the Sheppard and Enoch Pratt Hospital in Towson, Maryland (Bing, 1961, p. 170) (Figure 3-1). Both were actively corresponding with others around the country who were interest-

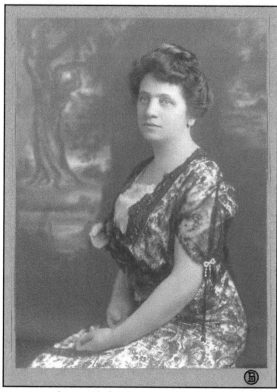

Figure 3-1. Eleanor Clarke Slagle circa 1914. (Reprinted with permission from the Research Library at the Fenimore Art Museum, Cooperstown, New York, John Davenport Clarke Papers, Coll. No. 12, Box 9, MWC.)

ed in the therapeutic use of occupation. Both Dr. Dunton and Mrs. Slagle saw a benefit in organizing these like-minded people to share ideas and experiences (Bing, 1961, pp. 176-177). Their aspirations to establish such an organization were temporarily put on hold when Mrs. Slagle resigned her position at the Henry Phipps Psychiatric Clinic on January 1, 1915 and returned to Chicago (Johns Hopkins Hospital, 1915, p. 57). Still, connected by their common interest and passion for occupation work, Mrs. Slagle and Dr. Dunton maintained their discussions through letters. They became lifelong professional colleagues and personal friends.

BACK TO CHICAGO

In the spring of 1915, the Illinois Society for Mental Hygiene funded the establishment of a community workshop, the Occupational Experiment Station, for patients with mental and physical disabilities. In keeping with the ideals of the Progressive Movement, the Mental Hygiene Movement, and the Arts and Crafts Movement the workshop was considered a laboratory where work activities were used to help those with disabilities adapt to community life. In establishing this workshop, the Illinois Society for Mental Hygiene hoped to gather data on social conditions that might contribute to mental illness and disseminate information that might help others in the pursuit of prevention of mental illness. Mrs. Slagle, already held in high regard by those in Chicago who were involved in the therapeutic use of occupation, was hired to establish the workshop. The workshop's patients, characterized by Mrs. Slagle as borderline mental cases and orthopedic cripples, were taught craft work such as knitting, rug weaving, basketry, tin work, ornamental cement work, cabinet making, and making wooden toys. Their handmade products were sold to the public—with part of the proceeds used to pay for materials and part of the proceeds paid to the patients, providing them an economic benefit, a feeling of self-sufficiency, and improved self-esteem (Slagle, n.d.; Slagle, 1919b; Thomson, 1917).

The Occupational Experiment Station also served as a school to train teachers to work in the workshop (Slagle, n.d.; Slagle, 1919b). Mrs. Slagle was very successful in expanding the services of the workshop and school—so successful in fact that additional space was needed (Thomson, 1917). In the fall of 1917, the Illinois Society for Mental Hygiene renamed the workshop and training school the Henry B. Favill School of Occupations to honor the beloved, late Dr. Favill who was instrumental in organizing the Illinois Society for Mental Hygiene (Favill, 1917, p. 87). The Henry B. Favill School of Occupations is recognized as the first school in the United States established for the training of occupational therapists.

Word of Mrs. Slagle's work and expertise in the therapeutic use of occupation was spreading. Soon other organizations sought her expertise in developing occupation and education departments. In the summer of 1916, she was given a leave of absence to complete summer courses in educational psychology at Columbia University in New York City with a particular emphasis on criminal psychology, mental hygiene, and hand work for defectives (Slagle, n.d.; Slagle, 1917a). That same summer, she spent one week completing a survey at the Montefiore Hospital and at the affiliated Country Sanitarium for Consumptives in New York at the request of their Board of Directors. Based on the results of her survey, she made recommendations for expansion of the department (Slagle, n.d.).

That same year, during her tenure at the Illinois Society of Mental Hygiene community workshop, Mrs. Slagle took an eight-week leave of absence from her position to "organize an occupational and educational department and work for a special group of defective criminals at Bedford Reformatory, Social Hygiene Laboratory" (Slagle, n.d.). The Laboratory of Social Hygiene at the New York State Reformatory for Women at Bedford Hills, New York provided treatment for psychopathic delinquent women (Spaulding, 1923, pp. 1, 14, 30-31). In a letter to Dr. William Rush Dunton, Mrs. Slagle wrote that her work at the reformatory "was one of the most interesting pieces of work it has ever been my privilege to do" (Slagle, 1917a). Mrs. Slagle equipped the department to teach courses in crafts including basketry, sewing, embroidery, knitting, crocheting, stenciling, painting, and carpentry. The patients participated in these crafts daily to use their energy and time constructively and earned the net profits from the sale of any article they made. During these craft sessions, the occupation teacher could observe patient behaviors such as ability to attend, distractibility, work preferences, ability to follow directions, and ability to learn in order to help with the patient's re-education (Spaulding, 1923, pp. 14, 30-31).

In 1917, while continuing her position as director of the Henry B. Favill workshop and training school, she was appointed General Superintendent of Occupational Therapy by the Illinois Department of Public Welfare. With the common interest of training occupational therapists, the Henry B. Favill School, the Illinois Society of Mental Hygiene, the CSCP, and the Illinois Department of Public Welfare joined forces to establish a training school. The training offered a five month comprehensive and rigorous course in curative occupations and recreation with the purpose of giving "instruction in habit training and occupations with special reference to the prevention and treatment of mental and nervous disorders" ("Training School," 1918, p. 635). Lectures were given at the CSCP while practical fieldwork experiences were provided at Elgin and Chicago State Hospitals (Chicago School of Civics and Philanthropy, 1917; Slagle, n.d., 1919a, pp. 29-30).

THE NATIONAL SOCIETY FOR THE PROMOTION OF OCCUPATIONAL THERAPY

By the second decade of the 20th century, many people were engaged in the therapeutic use of occupation with patients who suffered from mental illness, physical disabilities, and tuberculosis. Ideas and experiences were exchanged through articles published in professional journals such as *Modern Hospital, Trained Nurse and Hospital Review,* the *Maryland Psychiatric Quarterly;* through conference presentations; and through networking. Dr. William Rush Dunton Jr., Mrs. Slagle's friend and colleague from Towson, Maryland, continued to pursue the dream of organizing a national society of occupation workers. In 1914, he began corresponding with George Edward Barton, an architect and writer from Clifton Springs, New York. Mr. Barton became interested in the therapeutic use of occupations through his own illness experiences (partial amputation of his left foot and hysterical paralysis of his left side), and his efforts to heal himself to become a functioning member of society again (Andersen & Reed, 2017, pp. 21-23).

In early 1917, Dr. Dunton and Mr. Barton finally agreed on the initial framework of the new society and made a list of the people who would be invited to the inaugural meeting. Six people deemed to be experts in the nascent profession were invited. The invitees included George Edward Barton; Dr. William Rush Dunton, Jr.; Eleanor Clarke Slagle; Susan Cox Johnson, an arts and craft teacher on Blackwell's Island, New York; Thomas B. Kidner, an architect and vocational educator from Canada; and Susan E. Tracy, a nurse from Massachusetts. Mr. Barton decided to also extend an invitation to his secretary Isabel Newton, proclaiming that she should also be considered eligible for membership in the new society. The next year Isabel Newton became George Edward Barton's wife ("Barton-Newton", 1918). Arrangements were made for these founders to meet from March 15 to 17, 1917 at Consolation House, Mr. Barton's home in Clifton Springs, New York. Dr. Dunton, Susan Cox Johnson, Thomas Kidner, and Eleanor Clarke Slagle all arrived in Clifton Springs, New York by train, the main mode of transportation at the time. A prior commitment precluded Miss Tracy's attendance (Andersen & Reed, 2017, pp. 31, 37-39) (Figure 3-2).

At the meeting, the founders set about the business of forming the new organization agreeing on the name of the society—the National Society for the Promotion of Occupational Therapy (NSPOT). They established the organizational structure, adopted a constitution, elected officers and committee chairmen, and filled out an application to incorporate the new society (Newton, 1917). The founding vision for the new society, as stated in the constitution and the papers for incorporation, was consistent with the objectives of the progressive movement to embrace science and improve medical care for people. The vision stated was:

> The particular objects for which this corporation is formed are as follows: The advancement of occupation as a therapeutic measure; for the study of the effect of

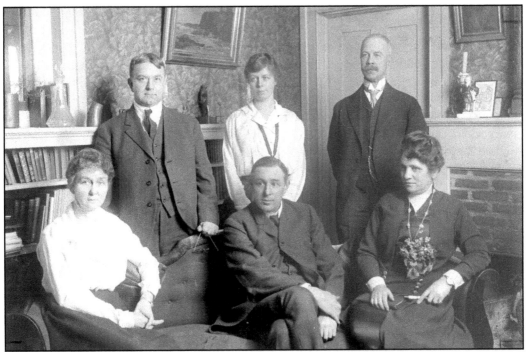

Figure 3-2. Founders of the National Society for the Promotion of Occupational Therapy. Bottom Row, left to right: Susan Cox Johnson, George Edward Barton, Eleanor Clarke Slagle. Top Row, left to right: Dr. William Rush Dunton Jr., Isabel Gladwin Newton, Thomas Bessell Kidner. (Reprinted with permission from the Archive of the American Occupational Therapy Association, Inc.)

occupation upon the human being; and for the scientific dispensation of this knowledge. (AOTA, 1967, p. 4)

In 1917, the use of arts and crafts was one of the primary modalities used by occupation workers. To distinguish this society and the new profession from other professions or workers, the founders stressed the importance and need for the therapeutic aspect of the use of occupation and the medical aspect of the use of arts and crafts, to separate itself from arts and crafts societies and arts and crafts teachers with no medical training (Andersen & Reed, 2017, p. 43).

Five of the attendees read papers at the founding meeting to share their experiences and ideas. Mrs. Slagle, Miss Johnson, Mr. Kidner, and Mr. Barton spoke about their work experiences, while Dr. Dunton shared information on the history of the therapeutic use of occupation. George Edward Barton was elected president of the new society and Eleanor Clarke Slagle was elected vice-president. Mrs. Slagle was also appointed chairperson of the Installations and Advice committee (Andersen & Reed, 2017, pp. 40-41). Her role as committee chair made her the face of the society as she was charged to "keep in touch with the changing conditions of institutions, to formulate methods by which Occupational Therapy may be introduced, and to confer with and advise any person or body desirous of investigating Occupational Therapy" (NSPOT, 1917, pp. 9-10). Taking this assignment to heart, through the next 20 years Mrs. Slagle participated in multiple life roles including volunteer leadership positions in NSPOT/AOTA, occupational therapy consultant to government and private agencies, administrative positions in state and private entities, and mentor to many.

As required by the constitution, Mrs. Slagle submitted a report on her activities at each annual meeting. She proved to be an excellent ambassador for occupational therapy. At the first annual meeting held six months after the founding meeting, Mrs. Slagle reported that she had received 60 letters requesting information about installing or organizing occupational therapy departments, gave 100 interviews on the work of occupational therapy, gave eight talks and class demonstrations on the hand work in occupational therapy, addressed an annual meeting of alienists (psychiatrists) and neurologists, and was preparing a course outline on occupational therapy methods to be instituted by the National Council of Defense and the National Red Cross (Slagle, 1917d, p. 28).

THE GREAT WAR

Three weeks after the founding meeting of NSPOT on April 6, 1917, America entered the Great War (World War I). As with all Americans and other professional groups, NSPOT was anxious to contribute to the war effort. In 1917, because of her association with Thomas Kidner (one of the NSPOT founders), Mrs. Slagle was invited by the Canadian Military Hospitals Commission to survey the work in their hospitals and make recommendations to extend occupational therapy services. While in Canada, Mrs. Slagle also made recommendations for a ward aides (occupation workers) program that was about to start at the University of Toronto (Slagle, n.d.).

Mrs. Slagle advocated for mobilization of forces for re-education of disabled soldiers who would inevitably return from the war in Europe ("Jobs for War Crippled Men, Is New Problem", 1917). Colonel Thomas W. Salmon, a psychiatrist, was charged with setting up a neuropsychiatric hospital in France for soldiers suffering from shell shock. He offered Mrs. Slagle the position in charge of re-education work with the overseas neuropsychiatric cases at this hospital, which was located 30 miles from the front lines (Andersen & Reed, 2017, p. 63). After careful consideration, Mrs. Slagle declined the offer believing that she would better serve by stimulating interest in training schools for occupation workers and providing services for returning soldiers in Chicago ("Aid to Invalids", 1917; Slagle, n.d.). She organized and conducted occupational therapy classes for the Chicago Chapter of the Red Cross, which eventually merged with the classes at the Henry B. Favill School. The majority of reconstruction aides in the Midwest were trained at this school under Mrs. Slagle's guidance (Lermit, 1921) and many of her students went on to start training schools in other parts of the country (Department of Public Welfare of Illinois, 1919, p. 63). Mrs. Slagle was particularly heartened by a training class that completed their training in November 1918. In a letter to William Rush Dunton she wrote, "... these classes are doing a wonderful amount of good spreading the gospel of Occupational Therapy" and "... the field is growing so rapidly and the need for the work being so definitely recognized that I think the outlook is entirely cheerful" (Slagle, 1918).

In addition to the schools in Chicago, Mrs. Slagle consulted on the establishment of two of the pioneer schools in occupational therapy. The first was the Philadelphia School of Occupational Therapy, where Mrs. Slagle delivered the opening address on October 2, 1918. The second was the St. Louis School of Occupational Therapy, where she consulted on the curriculum and gave the opening address on December 3, 1918. In that address, Mrs. Slagle advised the students that,

> ...the object of the work is to get the attention of a patient suffering from shell shock, hold it and then substitute a thought that will bring him to the execution of some work and give him employment... work is the normal medium that brings the joy of life" ("Plan for Curing Victims of Shell Shock Explained", 1918)

In 1918, she made a total of 78 addresses on the general subject of occupational therapy. That same year, the Surgeon General's office invited Mrs. Slagle to become a consultant in occupational therapy and pre-vocational work to the Department of Rehabilitation. Her activities with the Surgeon General's office drew the interest of people in England, Australia, and Canada (NSPOT, 1919a, pp. 27-28).

The Medical Department of the Army was aware of the success of the therapeutic use of occupation in reconstruction programs for soldiers in England, France, and Canada. The Medical Department of the Army wanted to establish similar programs to help with the re-education of disabled soldiers and sailors in the United States. To staff these programs the department created the position of Reconstruction Aide in Occupational Therapy (Andersen & Reed, 2017, pp. 55, 58). With the signing of the Armistice on November 11, 1918, soldiers started returning home from Europe. Those with disabilities and tuberculosis were sent to United States Army general, base, and camp hospitals for rehabilitation. The Medical Department of the United States Army sought Mrs. Slagle's expertise, appointing her supervisor of reconstruction aides in occupational therapy in December 1918. Mrs. Slagle was given a leave of absence from her work with the Illinois Department of Public Welfare to take the supervisory position with the Medical Department of the Army. In her role as Supervisor of Aides, Mrs. Slagle visited 21 of these hospitals.

Mrs. Slagle had to resign her position with the Medical Department of the Army in March 1919 due to a serious bout with influenza and pneumonia. She was one of the millions of people in the United States who became ill during the great flu pandemic of 1918. This virus spread throughout the United States and the world from 1918 to 1920 with more than 675,000 succumbing to the virus in the United States. The flu was particularly deadly for young adults, especially those serving in the military during World War I and the year after the end of the war. Fortunately, Mrs. Slagle recovered and was able to resume her position with the Illinois Department of Public Welfare and her work with NSPOT, including her public relations work ("Honor for Mrs. Slagle", 1919; Slagle, n.d.). Later in 1920, when the work of reconstruction of soldiers and oversight of the reconstruction aides in occupational therapy were transferred to the U.S. Public Health Service, Mrs. Slagle was appointed as a consultant to this agency (Slagle, n.d.).

In September 1919, during the third annual meeting of NSPOT in Chicago, Mrs. Slagle was elected president of the organization. She was the first woman elected president of NSPOT (NSPOT, 1919b, p. 36) and the only woman to serve as president until Winifred Kahmann, OTR (occupational therapist registered) was elected AOTA president in 1947. Nominated in 1920 for a second term, she lost by one vote to Dr. Herbert Hall (NSPOT, 1920, p. 26). She continued in her position as Chairperson of the Committee on Installations and Advice.

Planning the Next Chapter

In 1917, Mrs. Slagle wrote to her colleague, Dr. William Rush Dunton, about her desire to return to New York to be near her family. In her letter, she revealed that she was communicating with the New York State Hospital Commission about accepting a position with them, possibly as a vocational secretary; however, the challenges of the Great War (World War I) caused a delay in accepting such a position because of the changing personnel needs at her current position with the State of Illinois (Slagle, 1917b; Slagle, 1917c).

Eleanor had maintained a close relationship with her mother and helped her with her affairs after the death of her mother's second husband, Mr. Happ. He had become despondent over losing his job as a conductor with the Glenfield & Western Railroad and took his own life in June 1916 ("Lost Job on Railroad", 1916; "Suicide in Carthage", 1916). After Mr. Happ's death, and out of concern for her mother's well-being and health, Mrs. Slagle made frequent trips to Western New York to visit her mother until her mother passed away on January 5, 1920 following a lengthy illness ("Emma J. Happ", 1920). Mrs. Slagle took responsibility to sell her mother's house in West Carthage, New York ("Deeds Recorded At County Clerk's Office", 1920a, 1920b).

Her brother John had returned to New York several years before and purchased a house in Fraser, New York in 1917. The house, known as Arbor Hill, was located just west of Delhi, New York on the Delaware River and was built by Ebenezer Foote in 1797—a man who fought at the Battle of Bunker Hill and served General George Washington in the Revolutionary War. The house had many famous visitors, including Aaron Burr (famous for his duel with Alexander Hamilton) and Martin Van Buren (eighth President of the United States) (Lincoln, 1925). John's new home became the new Clarke Family homestead, a place where the Clarke family could gather for holidays and special events (Figure 3-3).

Mrs. Slagle was finally able to act on her desire to return to New York, although not initially for a position with the New York State Hospital Commission. She accepted the position of Executive Director of the New York State Occupational Therapy Society (also referred to as the Occupation Therapy Society of New York) (Slagle, n.d.; Lermit, 1921; Occupation Therapy Society of New York, 1921). In May 1920, Mrs. Slagle submitted her resignation letter to Charles H. Thorne, Director of the Illinois Department of Public Welfare (Thorne, 1920). The Illinois Society of Occupational Therapists gave her a farewell dinner on May 28, 1920 to honor all of her contributions to the state and to the profession ("Farewell Dinner for Mrs. Slagle", 1920). With Mrs. Slagle's departure to New York, the fate of the Henry B. Favill School of Occupations was sealed. The school had suffered some difficulties. No one was appointed to replace Mrs. Slagle and as a result, the Henry B. Favill School of Occupations was closed (Dunton, 1921).

It was a situation of the right person being in the right place at the right time. With changes in her personal life and changes in society, combined with her life in Chicago; her association with Jane Addams, Julia Lathrop, and other movers and shakers in Chicago; and her involvement with various women's organizations working for social and political reforms—these things all gave Mrs. Slagle a new purpose in life. Her observation of the benefit of participation in occupations for patients with mental illness and the suggestion of Julia Lathrop motivated her to enroll in the Occupations Course for Attendants for the Insane at the CSCP. This was the start of her career in occupational therapy. She was quickly recognized as an expert in the new field of occupational therapy and sought by many others

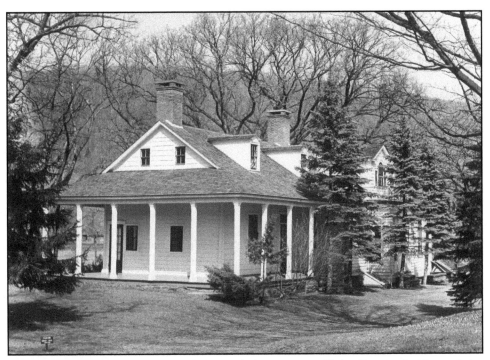

Figure 3-3. Arbor Hill in Fraser, New York, home of John Davenport Clarke. (Reprinted with permission from the Research Library at the Fenimore Art Museum, Cooperstown, New York, John Davenport Clarke Papers, Coll. No. 12, Box 7.)

seeking assistance to develop similar programs. Mrs. Slagle was hired and developed model occupational therapy programs at the Henry Phipps Psychiatric Clinic in Baltimore, at the Occupational Experiment Station in Chicago, and at the Henry B. Favill School in Chicago, the first training school for occupational therapists. Her efforts developing occupational therapy programs and occupational training schools was having a significant influence on the expansion of occupational therapy in the United States .

REFERENCES

Aid to invalids. (1917, December 29). Aid to invalids. Chicago woman confers in Washington on work here for victims of war's horrors. *Chicago Daily Tribune*, p. 5. Retrieved from www.newspapers.comAOTA. (1967). 50th Anniversary: Occupational therapy—Then… 1917 and now… 1967. American Occupational Therapy Association.

Andersen, L. T., & Reed, K. L. (2017). *The history of occupational therapy: The first century.* SLACK Incorporated.

Barton-Newton. (1918, May 9). Clifton Springs Press, p. 1. Retrieved from www.fultonhistory.com

Bing, R. K. (1961). *William Rush Dunton, Junior—American psychiatrist, a study in self* (Doctoral dissertation). University of Maryland. Available from ProQuest Dissertations and Theses database. UMI no. 6305931).

Chicago School of Civics and Philanthropy. (1909, July). *Announcements 1909 – 1910* (Bulletin, Volume 1, No. 1). Author. Retrieved from http://babel.hathitrust.org/cgi/pt?id=mdp.39015010775784;view=1up;seq=1

Chicago School of Civics and Philanthropy. (1911a, April). *Spring term courses, announcements for summer session.* (Bulletin 8). Author. Retrieved from http://babel.hathitrust.org/cgi/pt?id=mdp.39015010775784;view=1 up;seq=1 (which contains Bulletins 1-46, 1909-1920).

Chicago School of Civics and Philanthropy. (1911b, July). *Announcements 1911-1912 with register, 1910-1911.* (Bulletin 12). Author. Retrieved from http://babel.hathitrust.org/cgi/pt?id=mdp.39015010775784;view=1up;seq=1 (which contains Bulletins 1-46, 1909-1920).

Chicago School of Civics and Philanthropy. (1912, March). *Year book 1912-1913 with register, 1911-1912.* (Bulletin 15). Author. Retrieved from http://babel.hathitrust.org/cgi/pt?id=mdp.39015010775784;view=1up;seq=1 (which contains Bulletins 1-46, 1909-1920).

Chicago School of Civics and Philanthropy. (1917, December). Special course in curative occupations and recreation. In *Special Bulletin – Special Courses Curative Occupations and Recreation: Offered by The Chicago School of Civics and Philanthropy in Co-operation with the Henry B. Favill School of Occupations, Illinois Society for Mental Hygiene.* Author. Retrieved from https://babel.hathitrust.org/cgi/pt?id=hvd.32044079808143&view=1up&seq=25

Deeds Recorded at County Clerk's Office. (1920a, March 9). *Watertown Daily Times,* p. 6. Retrieved from www.genealogybank.com

Deeds Recorded at County Clerk's Office. (1920b, March 27). *Watertown Daily Times,* p. 7. Retrieved from www.genealogybank.com

Department of Public Welfare of Illinois. (1919). A conference of occupational therapy. *Institutional Quarterly, 10*(4), p. 63.

Dunton, W. R. (1921, April). The passing of the Henry B. Faville (sic) School. *Maryland Psychiatric Quarterly, 10*(4), 77-78.

Emma J. Happ. (1920, January 6). Emma J. Happ. *Watertown Daily Times,* p. 6. Retrieved from www.genealogybank.com

Farewell Dinner for Mrs. Slagle. (1920, May 28). Farewell Dinner for Mrs. Slagle. *Chicago Daily Tribune,* p. 19. Retrieved from www.newspapers.comFavill, J. (1917). Henry Baird Favill. Chicago: Privately Printed.

Former ticket agent at Nampa succumbs. (1933, October 1). *Idaho Statesman,* p. 3. Retrieved from www.genealogybank.com

Gertrude Slagle. (1986, April 22). *Idaho Press-Tribune,* no page number. Retrieved from www.ancestry.com

Honor for Mrs. Slagle. (1919, January 10). *Chicago Daily Tribune,* p. 15. Retrieved from www.newspapers.com

Illinois State Department of Public Welfare. (1939, June). Founder of occupational therapy work in Illinois. *Welfare Bulletin, 30*(5), p. 2.

Jobs for war crippled men, is new problem. (1917, July 13). *Chicago Daily Tribune,* p. 7. Retrieved from www.fultonhistory.com

Johns Hopkins Hospital. (1915). *Twenty-sixth report of the superintendent of The Johns Hopkins Hospital for the year ending January 31, 1915.* The Johns Hopkins Press.

Lermit, G. R. (1921, April). Vale. *Maryland Psychiatric Quarterly, 10*(4), 78-80.

Levine, R. E. (1987). Looking back: The influence of the Arts-and-Crafts movement on the professional status of occupational therapy. *American Journal of Occupational Therapy, 41*(4), 248–254.

Lincoln, F. H. (1925). Arbor Hill: 1791 – 1925., *The Walton Reporter,* June 6, 1925. (Brochure reprinted from this article available at the Research Library at the Fenimore Art Museum, Cooperstown, NY, in the John Davenport Clarke Papers, Collection 12, Box 7).

Lost job on railroad. (1916, June 15). *Journal and Republican and Lowville Times,* p. 7. Retrieved from www.fultonhistory.com

Meyer, A. (1922/1977). The philosophy of occupation therapy. *The American Journal of Occupational Therapy, 31*(10), 639-642. Reprinted from The Archives of Occupational Therapy, 1922, 1, pp. 1-10.

NSPOT. (1917). *Constitution of the National Society for the Promotion of Occupational Therapy.* Sheppard Hospital Press.

NSPOT. (1919a). Report of the Committee on Installations and advice. In *Proceedings of the Third Annual Meeting of the National Society for the Promotion of Occupational Therapy* (pp. 26-28). Sheppard and Enoch Pratt Hospital.

NSPOT. (1919b). Committees. In *Proceedings of the Third Annual Meeting of the National Society for the Promotion of Occupational Therapy* (p. 36). Sheppard and Enoch Pratt Hospital.

NSPOT. (1920). Report of the Nominating Committee. In *Proceedings of the Fourth Annual Meeting of the National Society for the Promotion of Occupational Therapy* (pp. 25-27). Spring Grove State Hospital and Sheppard and Enoch Pratt Hospital.

Newberry State Hospital. (1913). *Report of the Board of Trustees of the Newberry State Hospital for the period ending June 30, 1912.* Wynkoop Hallenbeck Crawford, State Printers.

Newton, I. G. (1917). Report of the secretary: Minutes of the first Consolation House Conference. *Proceedings of the First Annual Meeting of the National Society for the Promotion of Occupational Therapy* (pp. 19-23). Spring Grove Hospital Press.

Occupation Therapy Society of New York. (1921). *Brochure.* Occupation Therapy Society of New York. Archive of the American Occupational Therapy Association, Bethesda, MD.

Plan for curing victims of shell shock explained. (1918, December 4). *St. Louis Star and Times,* p. 7. Retrieved from www.newspapers.com

Peloquin, S. M. (1991). Occupational therapy service: Individual and collective understandings of the founders, part 2. *The American Journal of Occupational Therapy, 45*(8), 733-744.

Quiroga, V. A. M. (1995). *Occupational therapy: The first thirty years, 1900 to 1930.* American Occupational Therapy Association.

Slagle, E. C. (n.d.). *Experience of Eleanor Clarke Slagle.* Archives of the American Occupational Therapy Association.

Slagle, E. C. (1917a, January 17). *[Letter to W. R. Dunton].* Archive of the American Occupational Therapy Association, (Series 1, Box 3, Folder 23).

Slagle, E. C. (1917b, April 18). *[Letter to W. R. Dunton].* Archive of the American Occupational Therapy Association, (Series 1, Box 3, Folder 23).

Slagle, E. C. (1917c, July 10). *[Letter to W. R. Dunton].* Archive of the American Occupational Therapy Association, (Series 1, Box 3, Folder 23).

Slagle, E. C. (1917d). Report of the chairman of Committee on Installations & Advice: Minutes of the first Consolation House Conference. *Proceedings of the First Annual Meeting of the National Society for the Promotion of Occupational Therapy* (p. 28). Spring Grove Hospital Press.

Slagle, E. C. (1918, November 23). *[Letter to W. R. Dunton].* Archive of the American Occupational Therapy Association, (Series 1, Box 3, Folder 23).

Slagle, E. C. (1919a, September 30). Department of occupational therapy. *Institutional Quarterly, 10*(3), 29-32.

Slagle, E. C. (1919b, November 12). *Occupational therapy.* Proceedings of the Twentieth New York State Conference of Charities and Correction, Syracuse, NY. November 11-13, 1919. pp. 121-135.

Slagle, E. C. (1936). The past, present and future of occupational therapy in the State Department of Mental Hygiene. *Psychiatric Quarterly, 10*(1), 144-156.

Slagle, E. C. vs. Slagle, R. E. (1914, July 3). *Decree for divorce.* Circuit Court of Cook County. B 115.

Spaulding, E. R. (1923). *An experimental study of psychopathic delinquent women.* Rand McNally & Company for The Bureau of Social Hygiene.

Suicide in Carthage. (1916, June 9). *Utica Herald-Dispatch,* p. 18. Retrieved from www.fultonhistory.com

Thomson, E. E. (1917). Occupation and its relation to mental hygiene. *Modern Hospital, 8*(6), 397-398.

Thorne, C. H. (1920, May 17). *[Letter to E. C. Slagle].* Archive of the American Occupational Therapy Association, (Series 1, Box 24, Folder 161).

Training school for occupational therapists. (1918). Notes and comments. *Mental Hygiene, 2*(4), 635-636.

University of Chicago Library. (2010). *Guide to the Chicago School of Civics and Philanthropy: Records 1903-1922.* Retrieved from https://www.lib.uchicago.edu/e/scrc/findingaids/view.php?eadid=ICU.SPCL.CSCP

U.S. Census Bureau. (1910). *Washington County, Idaho, Weiser City, enumeration district (ED) 283, Image 1188, Sheet 2B, Line 74, household of William McBritney [sic], January 3, 1910.* Microfilm. Retrieved from http://familysearch.com.

U.S. Census Bureau. (1920). *Washington County, Idaho, City of Weiser, enumeration district (ED) 189, Image 1188, Sheet 1B, Line 95-97, household of Robert Slagle, January 3, 1920.* Microfilm. Retrieved from www.familysearch.org

World's greatest medical men here: To attend opening tomorrow of Henry Phipps Psychiatric Clinic. (1913, April 15). *The Evening Sun,* p. 2. Retrieved from www.newspapers.com

A Life Worthwhile

Living and Serving in New York State

"Only a life lived for others is a life worthwhile."
Albert Einstein

In June 1920, in what might be considered a homecoming, Mrs. Slagle moved back to New York State and took up residence in New York City. Hired by the Occupation Therapy Society of New York as the executive director, she was charged with the responsibility to lead the society's efforts to work towards the following objectives: 1) establish workshops and a training school for teachers of occupation therapy, 2) provide a registry of trained Occupation Aides, 3) assist hospitals and institutions to organize occupation therapy programs, 4) provide a sales department for products made by convalescents in occupation therapy programs, and 5) serve as clearinghouse for information (Occupation Therapy Society of New York, 1921). During Mrs. Slagle's tenure with the society and in pursuit of one of their objectives, she organized an Occupational Therapy Summer School at Byrdcliffe in Woodstock, New York, an artist colony in the Catskills. While Mrs. Slagle was not directly in charge of this program, which was considered by some to be postgraduate work, she did teach in the program. This program was only offered one time because of limited finance resources (Hall, 1921; House of Delegates, 1922, pp. 329-333).

Many of Mrs. Slagle's responsibilities with the Occupation Therapy Society of New York were similar to those she had with NSPOT. During the same time she was working for the Occupation Therapy Society of New York and volunteering with NSPOT, she served as a consultant in occupational therapy to the U.S. Public Health Service and as a consultant in occupational therapy to the National Tuberculosis Association (Slagle, n.d.-a). In July 1922, when her work with the Occupation Society of New York was completed, she was hired as the Director of Occupational Therapy by the New York State Hospital Commission.

Note: More information about Mrs. Slagle's activities and 20-year tenure in her position with the New York State Hospital Commission is provided in Chapter 5.

For the Good of the Association

"Do your bit now. Don't wait for the next opportunity."
Eleanor Clarke Slagle (Board of Management, 1931)

The name of the National Society for the Promotion of Occupational Therapy was changed to the American Occupational Therapy Association (AOTA) at the annual conference in 1921 ("American Occupational Therapy Association is new name", 1921). That same year Mrs. Slagle was elected Secretary-Treasurer of NSPOT/AOTA (NSPOT, 1922, p. 223), an office she held until 1937. Initially, as the Secretary-Treasurer Mrs. Slagle kept the association's documents in her kitchen and managed affairs from her apartment in New York City. In 1922, the Association established more formal headquarters, renting office space for $50/month in the Terminal Building at 370 Seventh Avenue in New York City (Kidner, 1926; "Report of Secretary-Treasurer", 1922, pp. 49-50).

Mrs. Slagle continued to handle membership applications, as well as providing information and advice about setting up clinical and educational occupational therapy programs, establishing state societies of occupational therapy, and hiring occupational therapists. The AOTA headquarters were moved to the Flatiron Building at 23rd Street and 5th Avenue in New York City in 1925. Although the rent for the office space, which also housed Mrs. Slagle's office with the New York State Hospital Commission, was $60 per month—$10 a month more than the rent at the previous building, the increased fee was justified by the convenience for Mrs. Slagle (Board of Management, 1926a; Kidner, 1926).

Mrs. Slagle categorized her work as Secretary-Treasurer as, 1) office work, and 2) work in the field. The office work involved giving advice on starting occupational therapy programs, such as advice on appropriate space, equipment and supplies needed, and hiring personnel. The general office work also included receiving annual dues, corresponding with members requesting information on establishing new state societies, and responding to other requests for information on topics related to occupational therapy (AOTA, 1923, p. 50-51).

In her roles as Secretary-Treasurer of the AOTA and as the Chairperson of the Installations and Advice Committee, local Junior Leagues sought advice from Mrs. Slagle to help establish and support occupational therapy programs in their local areas. The Junior League, an organization formed in the early 1900s as a volunteer organization to help cure social ills, supported establishment of facilities to meet the health care needs of children and adults. The support these local Junior Leagues provided to new occupational therapy programs often came in the form of financial support. Many of the relationships between these local Junior Leagues and occupational therapy programs continue today (Andersen & Reed, 2017, pp. 110-111; AOTA, 1923, p. 54; Board of Management, 1923; NSPOT, 1917, pp. 9-10; Slagle, 1930, pp. 385-386).

As part of her office work, Mrs. Slagle was also in charge of the association's placement service. The placement service assisted interested people to find jobs or schools to attend and, in some cases, to obtain scholarships to attend the schools. The placement service offered in the early 1920s was particularly time consuming, keeping lists of people seeking positions and also fulfilling institutional requests for these lists (Board of Management, 1925). Mrs. Slagle wanted to ensure the success of both the individual seeking a position and the hiring institution, so after careful consideration of the skills and abilities of the person seeking employment and the requirements of the position she would make her recommendation to ensure a good fit between employee and employer (Board of Management, 1926b, September 26). Mrs. Slagle's work in the field also involved giving public presentations and visiting institutions (AOTA, 1923, p. 50-51).

Setting Standards

As a founder and an officer of AOTA, Mrs. Slagle was instrumental in establishing its policies and procedures. In striving to promote professional recognition and improve professional status, she insisted on establishing and maintaining high educational and professional standards (AOTA, 1967). Soon after NSPOT was formed, the need to establish minimum standards of training for occupational therapists became a priority, especially since trained workers were needed to work with the soldiers disabled by injury or illness during World War I.

When the Medical Department of the Army established a new category of personnel in early 1918, Reconstruction Aides in Occupational Therapy, several programs to train Reconstruction Aides opened their doors. However, as no standards existed, training programs varied greatly as to content of courses, the length of the training, and the quality of the training. In an effort to secure qualified people, the Medical Department turned to the newly formed NSPOT for guidance. While NSPOT had started discussions on standards, minimum standards of training for occupational therapists had not yet been adopted. So, in the absence of formal standards, Mrs. Slagle met with the Surgeon General's office to provide guidance on this issue of training standards and schools that provided appropriate training for Reconstruction Aides.

At the second meeting held in New York City in September 1918, NSPOT began discussions on establishing training standards for occupational therapy workers. While Mrs. Slagle did not chair any of the committees tasked with establishing standards for training schools, she was very involved in the discussions and debates that occurred over a five year period of time (AOTA, 1922a, p. 76; AOTA, 1922b, p. 224; Johnson, 1918, 1919; NSPOT, 1920; "Round Table on Training Courses", 1923; Slagle, 1918, 1919).

Since Mrs. Slagle and Mr. Kidner worked together closely during the early years of the NSPOT, they developed a strong professional relationship and friendship. She was grateful for his guidance and support and even considered him a mentor (Clarke, 1932f). They would work closely over the next several years developing various mechanisms to ensure high standards for occupational therapists and to improve the professional status and recognition of occupational therapy by other medical professionals and the public.

Based on numerous discussions and debates in 1923, Mr. Kidner (President of the AOTA at that time), Mrs. Slagle, and Miss Ruth Wigglesworth (Chair of the committee developing uniform standards) worked together to develop a draft of *Minimum Standards for Courses of Training in Occupational Therapy*. These standards established prerequisites for admission including age and prior education, the length of the training program (which was set at not less than eight months of theoretical work and not less than three months of practical training), the content of theoretical coursework, and the types of practical training. Pushing their agenda with the Board of Managers and Association, the standards were finally approved by the AOTA membership in 1923 (AOTA, 1924). With passage of the standards, Mrs. Slagle became the main contact person at the Association overseeing implementation of the standards. She handled calls and correspondence requesting information about minimum

Figure 4-1. Mrs. Slagle's registration certificate from the AOTA. Note that she, as Secretary-Treasurer of the AOTA, is one of the signatories. (Reprinted with permission from the Research Library at the Fenimore Art Museum, Cooperstown, New York, John Davenport Clarke Papers, Coll. No. 12, Box 6, Folder 10.)

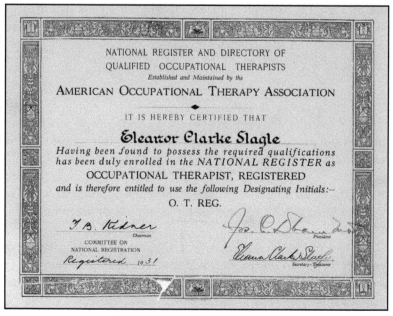

NATIONAL REGISTER AND DIRECTORY OF
QUALIFIED OCCUPATIONAL THERAPISTS
Established and Maintained by the
AMERICAN OCCUPATIONAL THERAPY ASSOCIATION

IT IS HEREBY CERTIFIED THAT

Eleanor Clarke Slagle

Having been found to possess the required qualifications has been duly enrolled in the NATIONAL REGISTER as
OCCUPATIONAL THERAPIST, REGISTERED
and is therefore entitled to use the following Designating Initials:—
O. T. REG.

COMMITTEE ON
NATIONAL REGISTRATION

standards for training schools and complaints about schools that did not meet the established standards. In cases where schools did not meet minimum standards, Mrs. Slagle brought the issue before the Board of Managers for discussion and guidance on how to handle the situation (Board of Management, 1925, 1927a, 1927b).

Although the association adopted *Minimum Standards for Courses of Training,* adherence to the standards was voluntary. To take it to the next level, Mr. Kidner turned his attention to developing a National Register of Occupational Therapists to provide a more effective mechanism to enforce standards and ensure qualifications of those calling themselves Occupational Therapists. The National Register, a list of those who met the training qualifications, would be provided to hospitals and institutions so they could hire qualified people (AOTA, 1932). Mr. Kidner appointed a committee to develop a proposal to establish a National Register, including a mechanism to inspect training schools and a process to add qualified graduates to the register. Mrs. Slagle was one of the people he appointed to the committee (Kidner, 1925).

Mr. Kidner was anxious to get a National Register in place, but the committee was slow to act. To move things along, Mrs. Slagle took the reins and researched methods and procedures used by other similar organizations with National Registers (Board of Management, 1927b, 1928). She then worked with Mr. Kidner to develop a proposal for a National Register. When a draft was completed, it was presented to the Board of Managers and the members. Eligibility for the register required graduation from a school that met the *Minimum Standards for Courses of Training* and one year of successful work after completing the approved training course (AOTA, 1932). For a period of three years after approval of the National Register, there was a mechanism to "grandfather in" or admit to the register, occupational therapists who (in lieu of completion of an approved training course) had significant experience working in the field (Board of Management, 1929a, 1929b). The plan for the National Register was approved by the membership at the Annual Meeting of the AOTA in 1929 (Kidner, 1930). Mrs. Slagle was eligible and admitted to the National Register based on her significant work experience (Figure 4-1).

Mrs. Slagle supported the association's next initiative to ensure high standards for Occupational Therapists. In 1931, Mr. Kidner requested the American Medical Association's Council on Medical Education and Hospitals (AMA-CMEH) take charge of inspection and accreditation of occupational therapy training courses. The oversight of this prestigious outside organization would bring increased legitimacy and status to the profession of occupational therapy. The standards developed by the AMA-CMEH, the *Essentials of an Acceptable School of Occupational Therapy,* were accepted in June 1935 and finalized in 1938, making the American Medical Association the accrediting body for occupational therapy schools (Report of the Council on Medical Education and Hospitals, 1935; Report on survey of occupational therapy schools, 1938).

PROMOTING OCCUPATIONAL THERAPY

Mrs. Slagle, was connected to the General Federation of Women's Clubs, a group aligned with the Progressive Movement objectives. Because of this she was often asked to speak to local, regional, and state affiliate clubs about the emerging field of occupational therapy. A few of the venues where she spoke and topics she spoke on included: The Chicago Women's Club—Occupational Education and Mental Therapy (June 1918); The Chicago Women's Club—Woman's Part in Teaching New Occupations to Wounded Soldiers (December 1918); and the Iowa Federation of Women's Clubs—Reconstruction Methods Applied to Our State Charges (May 1919; Club Notes, 1918; Downtown Clubs, 1918; Society, 1919).

After moving to New York State, Mrs. Slagle continued to deliver addresses and lectures to women's clubs and other organizations on the therapeutic use of occupation and reconstruction of patients with mental illness. She firmly believed that this was an excellent way to educate the public about occupational therapy programs in institutions and that audiences were eager to learn about the therapeutic programs (Slagle, 1924, p. 75). Some of the venues for her lectures included the Zonta Club of Buffalo, the Oneonta Rotary Club (in Oneonta, New York), as well as a number of clubs affiliated with the General Federation of Women's Clubs ("Chicago water withdrawal also assailed at Zonta luncheon", 1924; "Eleanor Clarke Slagle", 1925).

In 1920 Mrs. Slagle was named Chairperson of the Committee on Occupational Therapy of the General Federation of Women's Clubs, providing with her with increased visibility as an expert in the emerging field of occupational therapy. Many of the affiliated women's clubs invited her to speak about occupational therapy—giving her the opportunity to spread word of the benefits and successes of occupational therapy. The General Federation of Women's Clubs featured 50 state federations nationwide and a large number of affiliated local branches with more than three million members (Slagle, 1922, p. 81; Winslow, 1922, p. 10, p. 17).

One of the responsibilities of her position as Chairperson of the Committee on Occupational Therapy was to establish a means to educate women about the new field. The committee recommended 24 women to chair state federation's Committees on Occupational Therapy. These state federation chairpersons would then help educate state federations about occupational therapy. At the 1921 Biennial Conference of the General Federation of Women's Clubs held in Chautauqua, New York, Mrs. Slagle led a discussion on women's clubs influencing young women to take courses of instruction in occupational therapy to learn how to work with patients with mental illness and tuberculosis. The objective of the session was to bring together occupational therapy schools that had specific needs and the people from the

General Federation who could help schools meet those needs. At that same biennial meeting, Mrs. Slagle was able to secure space at the conference so that occupational therapy schools could meet with conference goers. This gave the schools the opportunity to talk about their specific programs and accomplishments and their specific needs, including money for scholarships and recruitment of students (Slagle, 1922, p. 81; "Timely Subjects Claiming Attention of Federation", 1922).

On several occasions Mrs. Slagle addressed meetings of the General Federation and affiliated women's clubs, such as the 1922 Biennial Session of the General Federation of Women's Clubs in Chautauqua, New York ("Timely Subjects Claiming Attention of Federation", 1922); the State Federation in Connecticut; and various New York State regional and local federation club meetings in Ogdensburg, Watertown, Poughkeepsie, and Long Island. Mrs. Slagle even had the opportunity to address the Woman's Civic Club of Hobart, New York (the local affiliate in her hometown), allowing her to reconnect with longtime friends and neighbors.

Archival newspapers and the handwritten minutes of the Woman's Civic Club of Hobart provide a record of these presentations. Her first opportunity to address the club came on September 17, 1921 at the home of Miss Elizabeth King who hosted the meeting ("Mrs. Slagle at Hobart", 1921). On May 27, 1932, Mrs. Frank Chappell hosted the meeting of the Woman's Civic Club of Hobart. Mrs. F. M. Lyon, President of the club, introduced Mrs. Ella Clark Slagle *[sic]* who then spoke to her hometown group about her work with the Rehabilitation Program of the State Department of Mental Hygiene. At the end of her presentation, Mrs. Walter Rich thanked Mrs. Slagle on behalf of the members, presenting her with a beautiful bouquet of roses (Minutes, 1932, p. 87). Lastly, on December 4, 1934 Mrs. A. L. O'Connor, President of the Woman's Civic Club of Hobart, presided over the club's business meeting at the New Hobart Hotel, the home of Mrs. James Aiken. Once the club's business was completed, Mrs. M. A. Damon, nee Mae Tennant, introduced her girlhood friend, Mrs. Eleanor Clark Slagle, who briefly described her work as Director of Occupational Therapy for New York State institutions. After the brief description of her work for New York State, Mrs. Slagle spoke about her lecture tour to Belgium and England where she had the opportunity to tour facilities for people with mental illness and to present two lectures about the New York State Department of Mental Health Occupational Therapy program. At the conclusion of her talk at the Woman's Civic Club, the club members gave Mrs. Slagle "a rising vote of thanks and … a corsage of gardenias" ("Civic Club Met at New Hobart", 1934; Minutes, 1934, pp. 19-20) (Figures 4-2 and 4-3).

INTERNATIONAL TRAVEL

Despite a busy schedule of work with the New York State Hospital Commission and her volunteer responsibilities with the AOTA, Mrs. Slagle occasionally found time for leisure pursuits, including foreign travel. After the very successful First Annual Institute and Conference of Chief Occupational Therapists, organized and presided over by Mrs. Slagle, Thomas B. Kidner wrote to Dr. William Rush Dunton:

> You will be glad to know that Mrs. Slagle has dropped everything and taken a trip to Bermuda with Miss Mary Shanklin. Mrs. Slagle's Institute last week was a great success, but between that and her other work she was nearly "all in," and I am very glad that she has gone away for a few days. (Kidner, 1924)

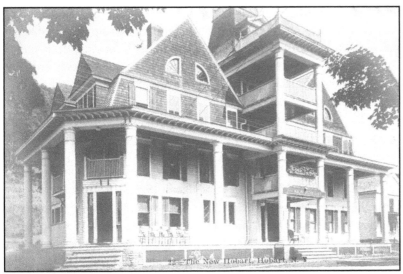

Figure 4-2. Old Postcard of the New Hobart Hotel. Reprinted with permission from the Hobart Historical Society, Hobart, New York. (Reprinted with permission of the Hobart Historical Society, Hobart, New York.)

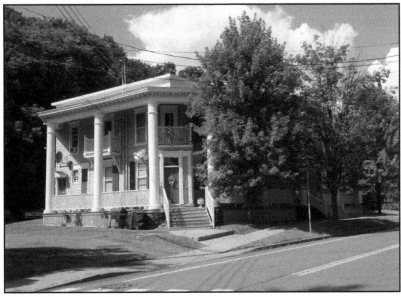

Figure 4-3. The former New Hobart Hotel circa 2018. Two upper floors were destroyed by a fire in May 1941 and removed. (© Lori T. Andersen. Reprinted with permission.)

Mrs. Slagle and Miss Shanklin set sail for Bermuda the last week in April 1924 for the two-day trip by sea to the island. They returned on the S.S. Fort Victoria, setting sail on May 3rd from Hamilton, Bermuda, and arriving back in New York on May 5th.

Two years later at Christmastime in 1926, in recognition and appreciation for her hard work for the AOTA, the Board of Directors presented Mrs. Slagle with a trip to Europe in the form of an $1100 foreign travel order from Thomas Cook & Son ("State Hospital", 1927). The travel grant funded the Mediterranean cruise that she took with her friends and colleagues, Dr. William Rush Dunton and Miss Mary Shanklin. One of Dr. Dunton's patients wanted to take a foreign trip believing it would be therapeutic for him. The patient asked Dr. Dunton to accompany him on the trip with the offer to pay Dr. Dunton's expenses, as well as an additional fee. Dr. Dunton did not want to go alone with the patient, so he asked Mrs. Slagle to go along. She was excited about this travel opportunity, and in turn asked her friend and colleague, Miss Mary Shanklin to accompany her (Bing, 1961, pp. 221-226).

The four of them boarded the R.M.S. Adriatic of the White Star Line in New York City on February 23, 1927 for a round trip cruise to the Mediterranean. During the days at sea, Dr. Dunton, Mrs. Slagle, and Miss Shanklin enjoyed the ship games, dancing, deck sports, lounging, and playing bridge. Once across the Atlantic they toured the ports of call, enjoying the shore tours at Madeira, Algiers, Monaco, Naples, Constantinople, Nazareth, Alexandria, Syracuse, and Gibraltar. In Egypt, they were thrilled to be able to see the Great Pyramids, the Sphinx, and King Tut's Tomb—all extremely popular tourist destinations at that time. Although Dr. Dunton's handwritten notes on the passenger list and cruise itinerary that he kept as souvenirs indicated the ship experienced rough seas and gale winds for part of their return trip home, they arrived home safely on April 11th after being away from home for nearly seven weeks (Bing, 1961, pp. 223-226; List of Passengers, 1927a, 1927b).

Scotland was Mrs. Slagle's next destination. In the summer of 1929, she accompanied Mrs. Elizabeth Harper, a client of her brother John Davenport Clarke, on a trip to Scotland. Mrs. Harper (nee Lizzie Burnie), emigrated to the United States in 1900 from her birthplace in Scotland and married her husband Walter shortly after her arrival in the United States (Petition for Citizenship of Elizabeth Harper, 1934). When Walter Harper passed away in February 1929, John Davenport Clarke thought a trip to her homeland would be beneficial for Mrs. Harper. Mrs. Slagle decided to travel to Scotland with her (Clarke, 1929e). While nothing is known about their activities while in Scotland, passenger lists indicate they sailed on the S.S. Caledonia from New York City on June 29th, arriving in Glasgow on July 7th. Their return trip, also on the S.S. Caledonia, left Glasgow on August 14th and arrived back in New York City on August 22nd (Arriving Passenger and Crew Lists (including Castle Garden and Ellis Island), 1820-1957, 2010; UK and Ireland, Incoming Passenger Lists, 1878-1960).

THE IMPORTANCE OF FAMILY

Eleanor and her brother John were very close. They supported each other's professional activities, helped each other in any way they could, and got together when time and circumstances allowed. When John purchased Arbor Hill in Fraser, New York it became the new Clarke Family homestead and gathering place for family and friends. Since Mrs. Slagle was living in New York City, she was able to visit with her brother John and the family more often than when she lived out of state (Clarke, 1931a, 1932g). Eleanor would take the train from Grand Central Station in New York City to Poughkeepsie, New York. There she would walk down a hill to the ferry station on the Hudson River. The ferry would cross over to Highland, New York where her brother or another driver would be waiting to drive her to Arbor Hill in Delaware County (Clarke, 1928j, 1931c).

In 1920, John Davenport Clarke threw his hat in the ring as a candidate for U.S. Congress from New York's 34th District. He was elected and began his first term in the Spring of 1921. Even though she was in Boston on April 11th to present at the First Annual Convention of Massachusetts Association for Occupational Therapy, Eleanor made time to send a congratulatory message to her brother ("Explain Therapy As Occupational: Leaders ...", 1921). The telegram read, "BEST WISHES FOR A SUCCESSFUL TERM (signed) PEGGIE". John would have known who the telegram was from as her close family called her Peggie and Aunt Peggie (Slagle, E. C. [Peggie] (1921). John was re-elected in 1922, but he lost re-election in 1924. He was not deterred. He ran again and was re-elected four more times: in 1926, 1928, 1930, and

1932. In Congress Clarke championed forestry, conservation, farmers, and dairymen's issues. His signature piece of legislation was the Clarke-McNary Act of 1924, a law that provided for public monies to reforest private lands.

John was quick to recognize the good work his sister was doing in the New York State Hospitals, both in private correspondence: "I have read with great care your report as Director of Occupational Therapy and must say I think it a splendid record of progress" (Clarke, 1928d), and publicly in the press. In one newspaper article, he sings her praises as a pioneer in her field who is now in charge of programs that help those with mental illness "make marvelous products" (Binghamton Press Bureau, 1928, p. 11).

In a letter from John to his sister Eleanor, he asks for information about her position with New York State, including current title, number of years of service, and current salary, so that he can speak to Governor Franklin Roosevelt on her behalf (Clarke, 1930b). One could speculate that John, in his position as a U.S. Congressman, was attempting to assist Eleanor receive a higher paygrade or salary increase for his sister. It is not known if John spoke with the governor or if Eleanor received a paygrade or salary increase at that time. However, records indicate that Eleanor was earning a salary of $4800 from New York State at the time of her death in 1942 (New York State Archives, 1894-1954).

Eleanor provided emotional support to John when he confided in her about his marital difficulties and the difficulties he had raising his son, John Duncan Clarke (Jack) (Clarke, 1928b, 1928k, 1929c). John provided Eleanor with advice about financial investments. Looking out for his sister, John offered suggestions on buying and selling specific stocks. In a letter dated November 5, 1928, he commented on the close call they had when the stock market took a downturn in the year prior to the stock market crash (Clarke, 1928i). The Great Depression in the 1930s was a difficult time for the country, including John Davenport Clarke. In efforts to reduce his expenses, he cut his son Jack's allowance, his wife Marian's allowance, some of his Arbor Hill employees pay, and even put some household items up for sale to make some money (Clarke, 1930e, 1931d, 1932a, 1933a). While in the past he had purchased items made by patients in occupational therapy classes to give as Christmas presents, he wrote to Eleanor in December 1931 stating, "Don't think I need any O. T. articles as I am cutting out most presents" (Clarke, 1931e).

In his congressional position, John Clarke was able to help some of Eleanor's occupational therapy colleagues who served as Reconstruction Aides. After World War I, the Reconstruction Aides formed an organization (the World War Reconstruction Aides Association) to preserve the history of their work, to maintain the friendships they had developed, and to advocate for themselves. The Reconstruction Aides were considered civilians working for the military, therefore they were not entitled to the same disability benefits as other military members who served. This changed in 1926 with the passage of the War Risk Amendments of 1926 that authorized compensation to women citizens, such as Reconstruction Aides, who suffered a disability during their service in World War I (Andersen & Reed, 2017, pp. 113-114; Public Law 69-448). When some of these reconstruction aides had difficulty receiving their due compensation, Eleanor contacted her brother, U.S. Congressman John Davenport Clarke, to seek his assistance to work with relevant federal agencies to ensure the Reconstruction Aides received the monies that they were entitled to (Clarke, 1929d; Slagle, 1929)

John looked after Eleanor's personal well-being and happiness as well. As he considered retirement from Congress, he mused about plans to spend his twilight years living at Arbor Hill close to his sister Eleanor. John offered Eleanor a piece of land at Arbor Hill, giving her choice of a number of prime sites. He indicated that once she chose a site, he would deed the land to her. Then, he advised, she might consider purchasing a house kit from Sears Roebuck and that his carpenter, Dan Ballantyne, could put the kit together for her (Clarke, 1928l, 1929g, 1931d). On occasion, John would send his sister Eleanor a gift of maple sugar cakes. Delaware County was well known for its maple sugar and Eleanor loved the cakes (Clarke, 1928c, 1929a, 1930c; Slagle, n.d.-b).

In 1928, to John Davenport Clarke's delight, his son John Duncan Clarke (Jack) followed in his father's footsteps and entered Brooklyn Law School in Brooklyn, NY (Clarke, 1928f, 1928g). With the elder Clarke spending most his time in Washington, D.C. serving in Congress, he asked his sister Eleanor, who was living in New York City, to watch over Jack (Clarke, 1928b). Jack was now in his early twenties, but he was not always acting in a responsible manner (Clarke, 1932d). He was a spendthrift with his father's money, charging items to his father's store accounts without his father's knowledge or permission. John tried, with limited success, to put constraints on Jack's spending (Clarke, 1929b, 1929h). John sought Eleanor's assistance, arranging to have Jack's law school bills to be sent to her. John then sent money to Eleanor to pay the law school bills and as well as additional money to pay for other things Jack needed (Clarke, 1928e; Clarke, 1928h).

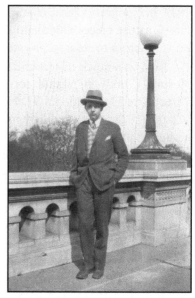

Figure 4-4. John Duncan Clarke ("Jack") in Washington, D.C., circa 1920s. (Reprinted with permission from the Research Library at the Fenimore Art Museum, Cooperstown, New York, John Davenport Clarke Papers, Coll. No. 12, Box 9, MWC.)

With Jack living in New York, Eleanor was able to keep an eye on his activities and report back to her brother (Clarke, 1928a). Jack often lost focus on his school work. He had a poor attendance record and failed a number of courses, which required him to retake those courses (Clarke, 1929e, 1929f, 1929i, 1930a). In an attempt to develop Jack's responsibility and appreciation for money, John paid him to do some work on legal cases and to write speeches for him (Clarke, 1930d, 1930f, 1931b, 1932b). Blessed with the musical talent of his Aunt Eleanor (aka Aunt Peggie), Jack also sang at weddings to earn money (Clarke, 1931c).

Jack graduated from law school in 1932 and was hired by Bond, Schoeneck, & King in Syracuse. Schoeneck, a former lieutenant governor of New York, was a friend of his father's (Clarke, 1932c, 1932e, 1933b) (Figure 4-4). With a new job and responsibilities, Jack began meeting his responsibilities and was ready to settle down. He met a young woman, Catherine Coville Odell, and married her on October 16, 1933 in the Sheldon Memorial Chapel of St. John's Episcopal Church in Delhi, New York. After the wedding the bride's aunts, Misses Elizabeth and Isabelle MacDonald, served a buffet luncheon for the couple and their guests at their country home near Delhi ("Congressman's Son Weds at Delhi", 1933). The couple was honeymooning on the shores of Otisco Lake in New York State when they were called home suddenly as Jack's father, the Congressman, was killed in a car crash on November 5, 1933 on his way home from a wedding ("Death of Clarke Ends Honeymoon Trip of His Son", 1933)

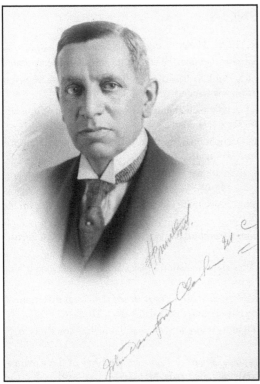

Figure 4-5. John Davenport Clarke. (Reprinted with permission from the Research Library at the Fenimore Art Museum, Cooperstown, New York, John Davenport Clarke Papers, Coll. No. 12, Box 7.)

(Figure 4-5). This was a very sad time for Eleanor, her sister-in-law Marian, and her nephew Jack.

After John's death, Eleanor maintained contact with her sister-in-law, Marian, who succeeded her husband in office (Figure 4-6). In March 1936, Eleanor celebrated with the Clarke family when her nephew Jack and his wife Catherine had a baby daughter (U.S. Census Bureau, 1940). A few years later, on March 6, 1939, she again grieved with the Clarke family when in a sad twist of fate John Duncan Clarke (Jack), was killed in a car crash ("Delhi Lawyer Killed", 1939).

For years, Mrs. Slagle was the face of the AOTA, and with 20 years of continual service as an officer of the association, she did more than any other founder to move the association and profession forward. With boundless energy, Mrs. Slagle was dedicated to spreading the gospel of occupational therapy. Through her presentations, she educated the public and other health care professionals so that they had a true understanding of occupational therapy. She developed an extensive network of long-lasting professional acquaintances, professional colleagues, and personal friendships. While she traveled internationally for business and pleasure, she remained a small town woman at heart from Hobart, New York, a family person who adored her brother John, her nephew Jack, his wife Catherine, and her grandniece.

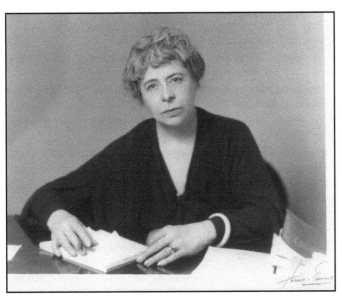

Figure 4-6. Marian Williams Clarke, wife of John Davenport Clarke and his successor in Congress. (Reprinted with permission from the Research Library at the Fenimore Art Museum, Cooperstown, New York, John Davenport Clarke Papers, Coll. No. 12, Box 7.)

REFERENCES

American Occupational Therapy Association is new name. (1921). *Modern Hospital, 17*(6), 554.

Andersen, L. T., & Reed, K. L. (2017). *The history of occupational therapy: The first century.* SLACK Incorporated.

Arriving Passenger and Crew Lists (including Castle Garden and Ellis Island), 1820-1957. (2010). *[database online].* Ancestry.com Operations, Inc., 2010. Retrieved from www.ancestry.com

AOTA. (1922a). The fifth annual meeting of the American Occupational Therapy Association: First day, morning session—October 20, 1921. *Archives of Occupational Therapy, 1*(1), 51-85.

AOTA. (1922b). The fifth annual meeting of the American Occupational Therapy Association: Third day, morning session—October 22, 1921. *Archives of Occupational Therapy, 1*(3), 221-230.

AOTA. (1923). The sixth annual meeting of the American Occupational Therapy Association: Morning session—September 26, 1922. *Archives of Occupational Therapy, 2*(1), 49-68.

AOTA. (1924). Minimum standards for courses of training in occupational therapy. *Archives of Occupational Therapy, 3*(4), 295-298.

AOTA. (1932). *1932 National directory of qualified occupational therapists enrolled in 1931 in the National Register.* American Occupational Therapy Association.

AOTA. (1967). Presidents of the American Occupational Therapy Association. *American Journal of Occupational Therapy, 21*(5), 290-298.

Bing, R. K. (1961). *William Rush Dunton, Junior—American psychiatrist, a study in self* (Doctoral dissertation). University of Maryland. Available from ProQuest Dissertations and Theses database. UMI no. 6305931).

Binghamton Press Bureau. (1928, May 19). Clarke Aided Fight in House for Hawes Bill. Binghamton Press, p. 11. Retrieved from www.fultonhistory.com

Board of Management. (1923, June 9). *Minutes of the meeting of Board of Managers.* Archives of the American Occupational Therapy Association (Series 3, Box 13, Folder 80), Bethesda, MD.

Board of Management. (1925, October 19). *Minutes of the meeting of Board of Managers.* Archives of the American Occupational Therapy Association (Series 3, Box 13, Folder 80), Bethesda, MD.

Board of Management. (1926a, September 26). Headquarters office. In *Minutes of the meeting of Board of Managers. Archives of the American Occupational Therapy Association* (Series 3, Box 13, Folder 81), Bethesda, MD.

Board of Management. (1926b, September 26). Placement service. In *Minutes of the meeting of Board of Managers. Archives of the American Occupational Therapy Association* (Series 3, Box 13, Folder 81), Bethesda, MD.

Board of Management. (1927a, May 19). *Minutes of the Board of Managers.* Archives of the American Occupational Therapy Association (Series 3, Box 13, Folder 81), Bethesda, MD.

Board of Management. (1927b, October 9). *Minutes of the Board of Managers.* Archives of the American Occupational Therapy Association (Series 3, Box 13, Folder 81), Bethesda, MD.

Board of Management. (1928, August 5). *Minutes of the Board of Managers.* Archives of the American Occupational Therapy Association (Series 3, Box 13, Folder 81), Bethesda, MD.

Board of Management. (1929a, January 7). *Minutes of the Board of Managers.* Archives of the American Occupational Therapy Association (Series 3, Box 13, Folder 81), Bethesda, MD.

Board of Management. (1929b, June 16). *Minutes of the Board of Managers.* Archives of the American Occupational Therapy Association (Series 3, Box 13, Folder 81), Bethesda, MD.

Board of Management. (1931, September 28). *Minutes of the Board of Managers.* Archives of the American Occupational Therapy Association (Series 3, Box 13, Folder 82), Bethesda, MD.

Chicago water withdrawal also assailed at Zonta luncheon. (1924, October 7). *Buffalo Evening News,* p. 18. Retrieved from www.fultonhistory.com

Civic Club Met at New Hobart. (1934, December 6). *Stamford Mirror Recorder,* p. 8. Retrieved from www.fultonhistory.com

Clarke, J. D. (1928a, February 22). *[Letter to J. Duncan Clarke].* Research Library at the Fenimore Art Museum (Collection 12, Box 3, Folder 19), Cooperstown, NY.

Clarke, J. D. (1928b, March 16). *[Letter to E. C. Slagle].* Research Library at the Fenimore Art Museum (Collection 12, Box 4, Folder 16), Cooperstown, NY.

Clarke, J. D. (1928c, March 22). *[Letter to John Duncan Clarke].* Research Library at the Fenimore Art Museum (Collection 12, Box 3, Folder 19), Cooperstown, NY.

Clarke, J. D. (1928d, July 25). *[Letter to E. C. Slagle]*. Research Library at the Fenimore Art Museum (Collection 12, Box 4, Folder 6), Cooperstown, NY.

Clarke, J. D. (1928e, September 22). *[Letter to E. L. Curnow]*. Research Library at the Fenimore Art Museum (Collection 12, Box 3, Folder 19), Cooperstown, NY.

Clarke, J. D. (1928f, October 1). *[Letter to E. C. Slagle]*. Research Library at the Fenimore Art Museum (Collection 12, Box 4, Folder 6), Cooperstown, NY.

Clarke, J. D. (1928g, October 3). *[Letter to E. C. Slagle]*. Research Library at the Fenimore Art Museum (Collection 12, Box 4, Folder 6), Cooperstown, NY.

Clarke, J. D. (1928h, October 31). *[Letter to E. C. Slagle]*. Research Library at the Fenimore Art Museum (Collection 12, Box 4, Folder 6), Cooperstown, NY.

Clarke, J. D. (1928i, November 5). *[Letter to E. C. Slagle]*. Research Library at the Fenimore Art Museum (Collection 12, Box 4, Folder 6), Cooperstown, NY.

Clarke, J. D. (1928j, November 22). *[Letter to J. Duncan Clarke]*. Research Library at the Fenimore Art Museum (Collection 12, Box 3, Folder 19), Cooperstown, NY.

Clarke, J. D. (1928k, December 7). *[Letter to E. C. Slagle]*. Research Library at the Fenimore Art Museum (Collection 12, Box 4, Folder 6), Cooperstown, NY.

Clarke, J. D. (1928l, December 27). *[Letter to E. C. Slagle]*. Research Library at the Fenimore Art Museum (Collection 12, Box 4, Folder 6), Cooperstown, NY.

Clarke, J. D. (1929a, January 2). *[Letter to A. J. Courtney & Son]*. Research Library at the Fenimore Art Museum (Collection 12, Box 3, Folder 18), Cooperstown, NY.

Clarke, J. D. (1929b, January 4). *[Letter to M. W. Clarke]*. Research Library at the Fenimore Art Museum (Collection 12, Box 3, Folder 20), Cooperstown, NY.

Clarke, J. D. (1929c, January 5). *[Letter to E. C. Slagle]*. Research Library at the Fenimore Art Museum (Collection 12, Box 4, Folder 6), Cooperstown, NY.

Clarke, J. D. (1929d, March 25). *[Letter to E. C. Slagle]*. Archive of the American Occupational Therapy Association. (Series 5, Box 24, Folder 161) Bethesda, MD.

Clarke, J. D. (1929e, May 8). *[Letter to E. C. Slagle]*. Research Library at the Fenimore Art Museum (Collection 12, Box 4, Folder 6), Cooperstown, NY.

Clarke, J. D. (1929f, June 11). *[Letter to M. W. Clarke]*. Research Library at the Fenimore Art Museum (Collection 12, Box 3, Folder 20), Cooperstown, NY.

Clarke, J. D. (1929g, November 8). *[Letter to E. C. Slagle]*. Research Library at the Fenimore Art Museum (Collection 12, Box 4, Folder 6), Cooperstown, NY.

Clarke, J. D. (1929h, December 13). *[Letter to E. C. Slagle]*. Research Library at the Fenimore Art Museum (Collection 12, Box 4, Folder 6), Cooperstown, NY.

Clarke, J. D. (1929i, December 13). *[Letter to M. W. Clarke]*. Research Library at the Fenimore Art Museum (Collection 12, Box 3, Folder 20), Cooperstown, NY.

Clarke, J. D. (1930a, January 8). *[Letter to D. E. Latham]*. Research Library at the Fenimore Art Museum (Collection 12, Box 3, Folder 19), Cooperstown, NY.

Clarke, J. D. (1930b, January 20). *[Letter to E. C. Slagle]*. Research Library at the Fenimore Art Museum (Collection 12, Box 4, Folder 6), Cooperstown, NY.

Clarke, J. D. (1930c, January 30). *[Letter to A. J. Courtney & Son]*. Research Library at the Fenimore Art Museum (Collection 12, Box 3, Folder 18), Cooperstown, NY.

Clarke, J. D. (1930d, April 17). *[Letter to J. Duncan Clarke]*. Research Library at the Fenimore Art Museum (Collection 12, Box 3, Folder 19), Cooperstown, NY.

Clarke, J. D. (1930e, March 31). *[Letter to M. W. Clarke]*. Research Library at the Fenimore Art Museum (Collection 12, Box 3, Folder 19), Cooperstown, NY.

Clarke, J. D. (1930f, November 13). *[Letter to E. C. Slagle]*. Research Library at the Fenimore Art Museum (Collection 12, Box 4, Folder 6), Cooperstown, NY.

Clarke, J. D. (1931a, January 2). *[Letter to Mrs. John Clemson]*. Research Library at the Fenimore Art Museum (Collection 12, Box 5, Folder 5), Cooperstown, NY.

Clarke, J. D. (1931b, April 17). *[Letter to J. Duncan Clarke]*. Research Library at the Fenimore Art Museum (Collection 12, Box 3, Folder 19), Cooperstown, NY.

Clarke, J. D. (1931c, May 18). [Letter to E. C. Slagle]. Research Library at the Fenimore Art Museum (Collection 12, Box 4, Folder 6), Cooperstown, NY.

Clarke, J. D. (1931d, August 12). [Letter to E. C. Slagle]. Research Library at the Fenimore Art Museum (Collection 12, Box 4, Folder 6), Cooperstown, NY.

Clarke, J. D. (1931e, December 4). [Letter to E. C. Slagle]. Research Library at the Fenimore Art Museum (Collection 12, Box 4, Folder 6), Cooperstown, NY.

Clarke, J. D. (1932a, January 7). [Letter to E. C. Slagle]. Research Library at the Fenimore Art Museum (Collection 12, Box 4, Folder 6), Cooperstown, NY.

Clarke, J. D. (1932b, March 1). [Letter to J. Duncan Clarke]. Research Library at the Fenimore Art Museum (Collection 12, Box 3, Folder 19), Cooperstown, NY.

Clarke, J. D. (1932c, May 16). [Letter to E. C. Slagle]. Research Library at the Fenimore Art Museum (Collection 12, Box 4, Folder 6), Cooperstown, NY.

Clarke, J. D. (1932d, June 4). [Letter to J. Duncan Clarke]. Research Library at the Fenimore Art Museum (Collection 12, Box 3, Folder 19), Cooperstown, NY.

Clarke, J. D. (1932e, June 8). [Letter to E. C. Slagle]. Research Library at the Fenimore Art Museum (Collection 12, Box 4, Folder 6), Cooperstown, NY.

Clarke, J. D. (1932f, June 24). [Letter to D. E. Latham] Research Library at the Fenimore Art Museum (Collection 12, Box 4, Folder 9), Cooperstown, NY.

Clarke, J. D. (1932g, December 9). [Letter to Mrs. Lewis Seymour]. Research Library at the Fenimore Art Museum (Collection 12, Box 6, Folder 1A), Cooperstown, NY.

Clarke, J. D. (1933a, June 5). [Letter to J. Duncan Clarke]. Research Library at the Fenimore Art Museum (Collection 12, Box 3, Folder 19), Cooperstown, NY.

Clarke, J. D. (1933b, August 18). [Letter to E. C. Slagle]. Research Library at the Fenimore Art Museum (Collection 12, Box 4, Folder 6), Cooperstown, NY.

Club Notes. (1918, June 19). Chicago Daily Tribune, p. 14. Retrieved from www.newspapers.com

Congressman's Son Weds at Delhi. (1933, October 18). The Freemans Journal, p. 8. Retrieved from http://nyshistoricnewspapers.org/lccn/sn83031249/1933-10-18/ed-1/seq-8/

Death of Clarke Ends Honeymoon Trip of His Son. (1933, November 6). Syracuse Journal, p. 2. Retrieved from www.fultonhistory.com

Delhi Lawyer Killed. (1939, March 16). Windham Journal, p. 2. Retrieved from www.fultonhistory.com

Downtown Clubs. (1918, December 8). Chicago Daily Tribune, p. 5. Retrieved from www.newspapers.com

Eleanor Clarke Slagle. (1925, October 8). The Oneonta Star, p. 5. Retrieved from www.newspapers.com

Explain therapy as occupational: Leaders show its important part in rebuilding soldiers. (1921, April 13). Boston Herald, p. 8. Retrieved from www.genealogybank.com

Hall, H. J. (1921). Occupational therapy in 1921. The Modern Hospital, 18(1), 61-63.

House of Delegates. (1922). Meeting of the Board Members and the House of Delegates of the American Occupational Therapy Association. Archives of Occupational Therapy, 1(4), 317-355.

Johnson, S. C. (1918). Educational aspects of occupational therapy. In Proceedings of the Second Annual Meeting of the National Society for the Promotion of Occupational Therapy (pp. 44-49). Sheppard and Enoch Pratt Hospital.

Johnson, S. C. (1919). Report of the Committee on Admissions & Positions. In Proceedings of the Third Annual Meeting of the National Society for the Promotion of Occupational Therapy (pp. 16-35). Sheppard and Enoch Pratt Hospital.

Kidner, T. B. (1924, May 2). [Letter to William Rush Dunton]. Archive of the American Occupational Therapy Association (Series 1, Box 2, Folder 19), Bethesda, MD.

Kidner, T. B. (1925, November 14). Memo: The members of the Board of Management. Archives of the American Occupational Therapy Association (Series 3, Box 13, Folder 80), Bethesda, MD.

Kidner, T. B. (1926, November 10). [Letter to William Rush Dunton]. Archive of the American Occupational Therapy Association (Series 1, Box 2, Folder 20), Bethesda, MD.

Kidner, T. B. (1930). The progress of occupational therapy. Occupational Therapy and Rehabilitation, 9, 221-224.

List of Passengers. (1927a, February 23). White Star Line—New York and Boston—Mediterranean Services [Brochure]. Archives of the American Occupational Therapy Association (Box 154, Folder 2105).

List of Passengers. (1927b, March 25). *White Star Line—S.S. Adriatic Passenger List. From Alexandria to New York [Brochure]*. Archives of the American Occupational Therapy Association (Box 154, Folder 2105).

Minutes. (1932, May 27). *Minutes of Woman's Civic Club. Secretary's Minute Book No 4: October 1929—June 1934*. Woman's Civic Club.

Minutes. (1934, December 4). *Minutes of Woman's Civic Club. Secretary's Minute Book No 5: September 1934—June 1937*. Woman's Civic Club.

Mrs. Slagle at Hobart. (1921, September 17). Mrs. Slagle at Hobart: All interested in Civic affairs invited to hear her today. *Oneonta Star*, p. 3. Retrieved from www.newspapers.com.

NSPOT. (1917). *Constitution of the National Society for the Promotion of Occupational Therapy*. Sheppard Hospital Press.

NSPOT. (1920). A general discussion on training of teachers. In *Proceedings of the Fourth Annual Meeting of the National Society for the Promotion of Occupational Therapy* (pp. 51-62). Spring Grove State Hospital and Sheppard and Enoch Pratt Hospital.

NSPOT. (1922). Third day, October 22, 1921, morning session. In Fifth Annual Meeting of the National Society for the Promotion of Occupational Therapy. *Archives of Occupational Therapy, 1*(3), 219-241.

New York State Archives. (1894-1954). *New York State Archives*. Albany, NY, USA; New York State Dept. of Civil Service, State Employee History Cards, 1894-1954; Series: 15029. Retrieved from www.ancestry.com

Occupation Therapy Society of New York. (1921). *Brochure*. Occupation Therapy Society of New York. Archive of the American Occupational Therapy Association, Bethesda, MD.

Petition for Citizenship of Elizabeth Harper. (1934, October 1). *Petitions for Naturalization from the U.S. District Court for the Southern District of New York, 1897-1944*. The National Archives and Records Administration; Washington, D.C.; Series: M1972; Roll: 925. Retrieved from www.ancestry.comPublic Law 69-448

Report of the Council on Medical Education and Hospitals. (1935). *Journal of the American Medical Association, 104*, 1631-1633.

Report of Secretary-Treasurer. (1922). Minutes of the Sixth Annual Meeting of the American Occupational Therapy Association. *Archives of Occupational Therapy, 2*(1), 49-59.

Report on survey of occupational therapy schools. (1938). *Journal of the American Medical Association, 110*, 979-981.

Round Table on Training Courses. (1923). *Archives of Occupational Therapy, 2*(2), 119-131.

Slagle, E. C. (n.d.-a). *Experience of Eleanor Clarke Slagle*. Archives of the American Occupational Therapy Association.

Slagle, E. C. (n.d.-b). *[Postcard to Mr. and Mrs. Happ— "Mother & Mr. Happ"]*. Research Library at the Fenimore Art Museum (Collection 12, Box 9, MWC), Cooperstown, NY.

Slagle, E. C. (1918). The training of teachers for occupational therapy. In *Proceedings of the Second Annual Meeting of the National Society for the Promotion of Occupational Therapy* (p. 53). Sheppard and Enoch Pratt Hospital.

Slagle, E. C. (1919). Report of the Committee on Installations & Advice. In *Proceedings of the Third Annual Meeting of the National Society for the Promotion of Occupational Therapy* (pp. 26-28). Sheppard and Enoch Pratt Hospital.

Slagle, E. C. [Peggie] (1921, April 11). *[Telegram to J. D. Clarke]*. Research Library at the Fenimore Art Museum (Collection 12, Series 3, Scrapbook 3), Cooperstown, NY.

Slagle, E. C. (1922). Report of committee on Installations and Advice. *Archives of Occupational Therapy, 1*(1), pp. 81-84.

Slagle, E. C. (1924). *Report of the director of occupational therapy* (pp. 71- 77). Thirty-fifth Annual Report of the State Hospital Commission. J. B. Lyon Company, Printers.

Slagle, E. C. (1929, February 15). *[Letter to J. D. Clarke]*. Archive of the American Occupational Therapy Association. (Series 5, Box 24, Folder 161) Bethesda, MD.

Slagle, E. C. (1930). Report of the secretary-treasurer. *Occupational Therapy and Rehabilitation, 9*(6), 379-393.

Society. (1919, June 4). *Quad-City Times*, p. 9. Retrieved from www.newspapers.com

State Hospital. (1927, March 10). *Gowanda Enterprise*, p. 1. Retrieved from www.fultonhistory.com

Timely Subjects Claiming Attention of Federation. (1922, June 24). *Jameston Evening Journal*, p. 5. Retrieved from www.fultonhistory.com

UK and Ireland, Incoming Passenger Lists. (1878-1960). *[database on-line]*. Ancestry.com Retrieved from www.ancestry.com

U.S. Census Bureau. (1940). *Delhi, County of Delaware, State of New York*. Line 4-6, May 4, 1940, p. 61. Microfilm. Retrieved from www.familysearch.org

Winslow, H. M. (1922). *Official Register and Directory of Women's Clubs in America*. Helen M. Winslow.

ENGAGED IN LIFE'S WORK

Working for the New York State Department of Mental Hygiene

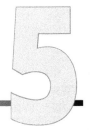

> *The aim of the work is to raise the level of human life of all sick, handicapped individuals in the hospitals of the service …. It is believed that carefully graded occupations, under medical supervision, suitably guided by adequately trained personnel, will continue to supply interests and exercises that serve to produce order in mind and body.*
>
> Eleanor Clarke Slagle (Slagle, 1933, p. 145)

Mrs. Slagle started her job as Director of Occupational Therapy with the New York State Hospital Commission on July 1, 1922. Her value to the State Hospital Commission of New York became evident early in her tenure when the Commission needed help to pass a bond issue. Compelled to act by a tragic fire at Manhattan State Hospital in 1923, the State Hospital Commission worked with New York Governor Al Smith and other interested organizations to pass a $50,000,000 bond issue for the purpose of enlarging and improving State Hospitals to provide for better safety, care, and treatment. Many of the buildings, built in the mid-1800s, were neglected through the years and in deplorable condition. The bond issue passed both houses of the New York State Legislature but, in accordance with the state's constitution, the bond needed to be approved by the voters of New York in a referendum (State Hospital Commission, 1925a).

The State Hospital Commission assigned Mrs. Slagle to work with other state officials on a publicity committee to garner support for the bond issue. For six weeks, Mrs. Slagle worked fulltime on this campaign. She was tasked with the responsibility to speak to women's organizations in the state to secure endorsements. Mrs. Slagle had already developed relationships with many of the organizations, their leaders, and their members through her active involvement in the General Federation of Women's Clubs. The targeted organizations included the Women's Christian Temperance Union (W. C. T. U.), the Eastern Star (affiliated with the Masonic Fraternity), the League of Women's Voters, and the New York State Federation of Women's Clubs. The New York State Federation of Women's Club, an affiliate of the General Federation of Women's clubs, was the largest women's organization in New York State with 578 local affiliates. Mrs. Slagle worked with the State Federation President, sending an official letter to all state members asking for their support for the bond issue. On

Election Day, November 6, 1924, the voters approved the bond issue by nearly a three to one margin (Slagle, 1925; State Hospital Commission, 1925a).

A Visionary Plan

Mrs. Slagle's first charge in her new role as Director of Occupational Therapy was to complete a general survey of occupational therapy in the State Hospitals and formulate a plan to extend occupational therapy services for the chronic, idle, and disturbed patients in the State Hospitals (The State Hospital Quarterly, 1922). While the State Hospitals primarily served patients with mental and nervous disorders, those with physical disorders such as orthopedic problems, tuberculosis, and blindness were also served (Slagle, 1936b). She made a total of 81 visits to the 13 hospitals in the State Hospital system during her first year to complete the general survey (Table 5-1). To improve and expand occupational therapy services in the State Hospital system, Mrs. Slagle worked to establish the administrative structure of the department, to promote the importance of occupational therapy in the system, and to develop the occupational therapy programs. She first secured qualified personnel to serve as Chief Occupational Therapists to assist in the development of occupational therapy programs. The special appropriation of $13,700 made by the New York State Legislature in 1922 to develop the occupational therapy programs in State Hospitals and to hire a Director of Occupational Therapy (Mrs. Slagle), also funded the salaries of these Chief Occupational Therapists.

After completing the survey of the occupational therapy programs in State Hospitals, Mrs. Slagle presented her vision of the whole scheme of occupational work in the State Hospitals to the State Hospital Commission. Using a wall chart as a visual aid, she presented the plan for occupational therapy services in the State Hospitals (Slagle, 1928, 1936b). The comprehensive plan defined the stages of occupational therapy work from treatment for the lower functioning patients who required considerable care, to treatment for the higher functioning patients returning to community living. In this plan, the stages were categorized as: 1) curative work, including occupational therapy and work in pre-industrial shops; 2) work in hospital industries; 3) sheltered employment; and 4) return to home and work in the community (Slagle, 1936b).

Curative work was provided on the ward or in occupational therapy centers for individuals and groups. This work included habit training, hand work, physical exercise, games, music, and recreation (Slagle, 1936b). Habit training, a program that Mrs. Slagle implemented years ago at the Henry Phipps Clinic in Baltimore, had patients follow established daily routines on an hourly schedule to create good habits of personal hygiene and maintaining cleanliness of the patient's surroundings (Slagle, 1928, 1936b). Patients participated in hand work, adapted craft activities on the wards, and, as they progressed, in centrally located occupational centers that offered an opportunity for a change in environment from the ward to bright, attractive workshops. The occupational centers encouraged re-socialization and participation in group activities. There were fewer constraints in the occupational center as compared to the wards, which helped to develop self-responsibility and self-respect.

Pre-industrial shops (also considered curative work) were designed to further the readjustment of patients to normal environments. In these shops, a patient's aptitude for certain work could be evaluated as the patient received basic training for various types of industrial work. Book binding, printing, making willow furniture, and cement work—making blocks,

TABLE 5-1. DEPARTMENT OF MENTAL HYGIENE— STATE HOSPITALS/SCHOOLS*	
At the Start of Mrs. Slagle's Tenure	**Added Since the Start of Mrs. Slagle's Tenure**
Binghamton State Hospital	Creedmoor State Hospital
Brooklyn State Hospital	Harlem Valley State Hospital
Buffalo State Hospital	Marcy State Hospital
Central Islip State Hospital	Pilgrim State Hospital
Gowanda State Hospital	Psychiatric Institute and Hospital
Hudson River State Hospital	Rockland State Hospital
King's Park State Hospital	Syracuse Psychiatric Hospital
Manhattan State Hospital	Craig Colony for Epileptics
Middletown State Homeopathic Hospital	Letchworth Village
Rochester State Hospital	Newark State School
St Lawrence State Hospital	Rome State School
Utica State Hospital	Syracuse State School
Willard State Hospital	Wassaic State School

*State Hospitals/Schools administered by the State Hospital Commission/Department of Mental Hygiene at the start and end of Eleanor Clarke Slagle's tenure (1922 to 1942).

benches, bird baths, and urns out of cement—were some activities in the pre-industrial shops (Slagle, 1928; Slagle, 1936b).

As a patient became more productive in the pre-industrial shops and gradually spent less and less time participating in physical exercises, games, and recreation, they were referred to work in hospital industries. The hospital industries included taking care of buildings and grounds, working in workshops, working in farms and gardens, and/or providing indoor service. As a step toward parole (discharge home), patients would be assigned to work in sheltered workshops under the supervision of a physician and, if appropriate, returned home to work in the community (Slagle, 1936b).

The commission approved the plan and with great enthusiasm Mrs. Slagle set about her work to achieve her vision of developing a premier occupational therapy department. She was guided by her general plan of a comprehensive occupational therapy program in the State Hospitals, and her "… firm and abiding conviction, formed after many years of experience, that occupational therapy, properly administered and applied, will bring more happy and abundant lives to those committed to the care of the State in its great hospital system" (Slagle, 1924, p. 77). Politically astute, Mrs. Slagle was able to convince the commissioners to support the occupational therapy programs (Cromwell, 1977) (Figure 5-1).

Mrs. Slagle strongly believed in the need for a proper prescription from a physician and documentation of the patient's response to occupational therapy treatment to communicate with the physician, in part because it was a means to educate physicians about occupational therapy. While physicians wouldn't necessarily be able to prescribe a specific occupation for a patient, the physician could prescribe "the kind of occupation needed, such as stimulating, sedative, mechanical, intellectual, academic or varied. If special movements are to be involved, as in orthopedic cases, ..." (Slagle, 1921, p. 45), then trained and qualified Occupational Therapists would be able to carefully select appropriate activities, adapt the activities, and grade the effort required to participate in the activity to ensure successful treatment (Slagle, 1930). The Occupational Therapist could then report back a patient's reaction to the prescribed work such as mental, emotional, and fatigue levels (Slagle, 1921). Physicians who understood the purpose and value of occupational therapy would support the programs and refer

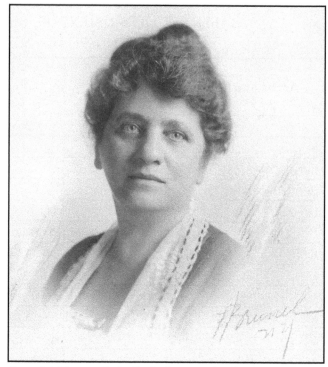

Figure 5-1. Eleanor Clarke Slagle. (Reprinted with permission of the Research Library at the Fenimore Art Museum, Cooperstown, New York, John Davenport Clarke Papers, Coll. No. 12, Box 7.)

patients for treatment, thereby helping to expand the services in the State Hospital system (Occupational Therapy Notes, 1925; Slagle, 1921).

To set her plan in motion, Mrs. Slagle requested the commission grant her permission to hire three employees to work under her direction. First was a stenographic service to assist with correspondence, reports, and memos to ensure a permanent record of such activities. Second was a supervisor to develop graded work projects in the various hospitals. And third was a supervisor to organize a physical education and recreation program (Slagle, 1924). In 1927, Harriet A. Robeson was hired as Assistant Director to help with developing programs in the various hospitals and in 1924, James E. Simpson was hired to supervise the physical training and recreation programs in the State Hospitals (Slagle, 1926)

Early in Mrs. Slagle's efforts to develop the statewide occupational therapy programs, she worked to determine the specific needs in each institution and to obtain more space for the programs. Additionally, she set up self-improvement or training classes for attendants assigned to work in occupational therapy programs (Slagle, 1924). The expansion of habit training programs for lower level patients showed the most progress and success, as this program could be easily established and implemented on the wards (Slagle, 1925, 1928, 1929). Progress in establishing pre-industrial work programs was slower and uneven in the various institutions, in part because of the need to first obtain materials, equipment, space for shops, and qualified people to run these programs. Search for suitable shop space continued through the years, with Mrs. Slagle adamant that basement space was not suitable (Slagle, 1926, 1928, 1938, 1940).

The pre-industrial programs included willow crafts, usually making willow baskets and willow furniture. Mrs. Slagle had first learned willow crafts during her time working for the Department of Public Welfare in Illinois. Limited funds to purchase materials for patients to use during the Great War and immediately after inspired Occupational Therapists to find no cost to low-cost materials for patient treatment. Waste materials and salvage materials were often used, and in the case of willow furniture, the willow was grown and harvested by the patients as part of their treatment. Mrs. Slagle had completed an extensive analysis of every step in the process from planting to completing a willow product. Patients skills and abilities were matched to a specific step in the process such as planting, harvesting, and/or preparing the willow rods, and constructing the piece of furniture. The finished product was frequently used around the institution, giving a sense of pride to the patients engaged in making the products. It was also a cost savings for the institutions since new furniture did not need to be purchased. There was a similar benefit in offering cement work in the pre-industrial programs (AOTA, 1924; Slagle, 1935, 1937, 1940).

Patients in occupational therapy classes at St. Lawrence State Hospital helped create and maintain a bird sanctuary, including building birdhouses and feeding platforms. Patients in occupational therapy also developed and maintained a sunken garden and flower gardens as part of the program at St. Lawrence State Hospital. Additionally, library services in some institutions were slowly transferred to occupational therapy since reading was considered an occupation for patients that had therapeutic benefit. To help with operation of the library, patients participated in book binding and book repair services (Slagle, 1935, 1937).

Physical Training and Recreation

Lack of physical and social activity in institutions was seen as physically and mentally detrimental to the patients. Therefore, the physical training and recreation program was established to provide for a balance in life that would include work, play, and physical fitness activities to overcome the negative effects of idleness (Slagle, 1933). James E. Simpson was appointed to the position of supervisor of physical education on November 3, 1924 to oversee all physical training and recreation activities under the direction of the Director of Occupational Therapy (Slagle, 1926). Carefully graded and adapted physical exercises, in the form of active sports and games, enabled patients of all endurance levels to participate (Slagle, 1927, 1928). Recreational activities, both passive and active, were offered to help with physical and/or social rehabilitation. Entertainment such as moving pictures, concerts, community singing, folk dances, victrolas, and radios were offered to engage the patients. As Mr. Simpson developed the program, efforts focused on development of playfields and acquiring recreational equipment. Field Days on the new playfields became highly anticipated annual events (Slagle, 1927, 1930; Anderson, 1931; "Fourth of July Celebrated at State Hospital", 1932; "Hospital Here to Have Field Day on June 7", 1934; "Marcy Field Day Viewed by 2,200", 1935).

Aware of the State's concerns about financial aspects of programs, the Bureau of Occupational Therapy took steps to control costs, from using waste materials to create craft projects to using funds raised by selling surplus articles made in occupational therapy treatment classes to purchase recreational equipment (Slagle, 1928). During the Great Depression, a time of significant economic stress for the country, Mrs. Slagle arranged with the Temporary Employment Relief Administration, a New York State Program, and with the

Civil Works Administration of New York City to entertain patients with fine concerts given by experienced musicians. Over the course of a couple of years, the musical units presented a total of 137 programs to Brooklyn State Hospital, Manhattan State Hospital, Rockland State Hospital, and the Psychiatric Institute and Hospital (Slagle, 1934a, 1935).

Mrs. Slagle always pushed for highly trained, qualified professionals to implement programs, including physical training and recreation programs. Pointing out the benefit of physical development and correctional exercise, Mrs. Slagle stated,

> … correctional phase should only be undertaken by the thoroughly trained, qualified instructor who has had sufficient education and training along these special lines to know that such exercises as the physician may prescribe are the only ones to be tried, and it is realized that to co-operate fully is highly important and necessary … Untrained workers lack the ability to plan ahead; they have no theoretical appreciation or objective. (Slagle, 1937, p. 136)

Word of success of the physical training and recreation programs spread. Many institutions wanted to develop similar programs and requested information about the different games and programs used by the New York State Hospitals. To satisfy the requests for information, Mrs. Slagle authored a book titled *Games and Field Day Programs*. More than 250 games and activities used to engage patients in the programs, including adaptations to enable the patients of different abilities to participate, were described in the book. Printed and bound by the Central Islip State Hospital Occupational Therapy Print Shop, the book was in great demand and received favorable reviews (Slagle, 1933, 1934b).

In the early years, Mrs. Slagle's efforts focused on securing qualified personnel and she personally recruited Occupational Therapists to fill vacant positions. To meet the needs of the State Hospital system for highly qualified personnel, Mrs. Slagle expressed a desire to establish a training school for Occupational Therapists, since New York State did not have any such programs. In anticipation of starting a program, Mrs. Slagle began working on a syllabus for undergraduate and post-graduate programs (Slagle, 1924, 1926). In 1928, knowing of Mrs. Slagle's desire to establish a school in New York State and always supportive of his sister, John Davenport Clarke wrote to her about the possibility of purchasing the Sheldon Estate in Delhi, New York so her National Association could establish an occupational therapy school on the property. The Sheldon Estate was located on the land where the Delaware Academy in Delhi, New York is now located. John suggested that she and Mr. Thomas Kidner (President of the AOTA at that time) come to look at the property. If she wanted to purchase the estate, he of course would back the project (Clarke, 1928). Nothing came from the suggestion and the estate was later purchased by Delaware Academy.

Reorganization and A New Name—Department of Mental Hygiene

A change in the organization of the New York State government combined the State Hospital Commission and State Commission for Mental Defectives, creating the New York State Department of Mental Hygiene effective January 1, 1927. This newly formed Department of Mental Hygiene was now responsible for administration of institutions formerly under the State Hospital Commission. The Department of Occupational Therapy, now part of the Department of Mental Hygiene, was renamed the Bureau of Occupational Therapy (Department of Mental Hygiene, 1928a).

A few years later, the Commissioner of Mental Hygiene suggested that Mrs. Slagle work with an official of New York University to develop a training course in occupational therapy (Slagle, 1930). It wasn't until years later in 1941 that New York University opened an occupational therapy program. The new program was headed by Susan C. Wilson, OTR, the Chief Occupational Therapist at Brooklyn State Hospital, one of the hospitals in the Department of Mental Hygiene system. Mrs. Slagle consulted on the curriculum development of the New York University program. Columbia University also opened a program in New York City in 1941 under the direction of Marjorie Fish, OTR. Ms. Fish later became an Executive Director of the AOTA (Slagle, 1942).

SYLLABUS FOR TRAINING OF NURSES IN OCCUPATIONAL THERAPY

Mrs. Slagle believed that education of nursing staff was an important part of promoting occupational therapy services, as nurses who understood the purpose of occupational therapy would embrace the services and occasionally assist in providing the services (Slagle, 1921, 1925, 1926). To meet this objective, Mrs. Slagle prepared a syllabus for use in nurses' training schools in New York State Hospitals to educate student nurses in the practical and theoretical aspects of occupational therapy. As stated by Mrs. Slagle:

> The object has not been to make them occupational therapists, but to acquaint them thoroughly with the aims and methods of this newer arm of the medical service and, above all, to give them an understanding of the necessity and value of occupational therapy in the treatment of mental patients. (Slagle, 1925, p. 84)

The syllabus, continually tweaked through the years, outlined a training course that consisted of six one-hour lectures on such topics as history of OT, methods and practice, habit training, use of handcrafts, and physical training and recreation; as well as 10 two-hour sessions making handicrafts such as knitting, making baskets, making rugs, and woodworking, with an emphasis on using waste material to make crafts (Slagle & Robeson, 1941). During the first year, 153 nurses received this instruction (Slagle, 1925). By 1937, 1550 nurses had received the training.

After several years of tweaking the syllabus, and because of numerous requests from other states and countries seeking to develop similar programs, the *Syllabus for Training of Nurses in Occupational Therapy* was published in the early 1930s (Slagle, 1931). The book, a collaboration between Mrs. Slagle and Miss Harriet Robeson, was printed by the State Hospitals Press in Utica, New York. Requests for copies of the syllabus continued through the years (Slagle, 1938). A second edition was published in 1941 (Slagle & Robeson, 1941).

ANNUAL INSTITUTE FOR CHIEF OCCUPATIONAL THERAPISTS

Mrs. Slagle understood that part of improving and expanding occupational therapy programs in the State Hospital system required developing the knowledge and skills of the occupational therapy personnel. Developing a cohesive group, a team that could share needs, problems, and solutions was also an important part of improving and expanding occupational therapy programs (Slagle, 1925). To "further the medical, technical, and practical instruction of those engaged in the service" (Occupational Therapy Notes, 1925, p. 300), Mrs. Slagle decided to organize an institute for Chief Occupational Therapists. The Institute for Chief Occupational Therapists had the additional objectives of promoting the occupational therapy work in the State Hospitals and mentoring of the occupational therapy personnel.

In organizing the first institute, held from April 21 to 24, 1924 in the State Hospital Commission office (State Hospital Commission, 1925b, p. 41), Mrs. Slagle enlisted several groups of people directly interested in the occupational therapy work in the State Hospitals, including members of the Hospital Commission, hospital superintendents, inspectors, and occupational therapy personnel. Many of these people gave addresses, papers, and/or demonstrations of crafts. As part of mentoring the Chief Occupational Therapists, Mrs. Slagle assigned presentation topics to each of the Chief Occupational Therapists for the first institute (Slagle, 1926). By participating in the institute, these Occupational Therapists gained hope for the future, a sense of personal responsibility for lifelong learning, courage, and the desire to try and verify results of new methods and occupations for patient care (Slagle, 1925).

With the outstanding success of the first institute, Mrs. Slagle requested the State Hospital Commission to support the establishment of an Annual Institute (Slagle, 1925a). Her request was approved (Slagle, 1926). A total of 15 Annual Institutes for Chief Occupational Therapists were held from 1924 to 1942. Economic reasons, caused in part by the Great Depression, precluded holding an Annual Institute in 1934 and again in 1936. The annual institutes were recessed again in 1939 and 1940.

Mrs. Slagle organized and presided over each Annual Institute. The topics presented were varied, focusing on the medical aspects of occupational therapy and the technical and social aspects to address the interests and training needs of the Chief Occupational Therapists (Slagle, 1925). Addresses, papers, and practical demonstrations of arts and craft activities were all part of the Annual Institutes. The institutes featured talks and demonstrations on block printing, working with hand wrought iron, weaving tapestries, antique quilts, Central European arts and crafts, and using puppets and marionettes in therapy. Frequently site visits to the different state institutions were included as part of the institute so attendees could learn about the programs and resources at the other institutions. During these visits, Mrs. Slagle often served as the tour guide, or the cicerone as she called herself, showing off the individual occupational therapy departments that were under her direction ("Annual Institute of Occupational Therapists", 1930). She commented that these multiple visits during a scheduled institute "took the form of a traveling seminar" (Department of Mental Hygiene, 1934, p. 74). Recognizing educational, social, and cultural contributions of museums, museum visits became a feature of some of the institutes in the late 1920s and early 1930s ("Annual Institute of Occupational Therapists", 1930; Slagle, 1930).

The seventh Annual Institute of Chief Occupational Therapists in 1930 offered a very special visit to Val-kill Industries in Hyde Park, New York. Val-kill Industries was a business venture of Mrs. Franklin D. Roosevelt and some of her friends. Val-kill was known for making furniture and for its metal forge that made pewter objects. After touring the workshop to see these crafts made, the attendees were treated to a tea at the Roosevelt home ("Annual Institute of Occupational Therapists", 1930; Department of Mental Hygiene, 1931; Slagle, 1931). At the time of this Institute, Franklin D. Roosevelt was serving as governor of New

York State and Mrs. Roosevelt as First Lady of New York State. Governor Roosevelt was elected President of the United States in 1932 and Mrs. Roosevelt became First Lady of the United States when her husband was sworn into office in March 1933.

The success and reputation of the Annual Institutes for Chief Occupational Therapists spread. Attendance at the institutes was restricted to State Hospital/Department of Mental Hygiene personnel, but despite this many outsiders requested permission to attend and occasionally some lucky ones were able to secure an invitation (Slagle, 1930). Mrs. Slagle organized and presided over her last Annual Institute for Chief Occupational Therapists, the 15th Institute, from April 27 to 29, 1942 at the Psychiatric Institute and Hospital in New York City where she had an office (Department of Mental Hygiene, 1943a).

ANNUAL NEW YORK STATE FAIR EXHIBIT

The New York State Fair was held every year in late August, early September in Syracuse, New York. As with many state and county fairs, along with the contests and entertainment there were numerous exhibits presented by various organizations. In 1841, New York State was the first state to hold a state fair (New York State, 2020). The Department of Occupational Therapy, headed by Mrs. Slagle, first displayed articles created by occupational therapy patients at the New York State Fair in 1922. In her first annual report, Mrs. Slagle indicated that she was already planning to introduce other interesting features to the occupational therapy exhibit in 1923 to educate the public on the value of occupational therapy. With each yearly exhibit, she believed it was important to exhibit the newer features of treatment through creating simple, interesting exhibits with visual appeal (Slagle, 1924, 1935).

Subsequent state fair exhibits included demonstrations of the arts and crafts activities used in occupational therapy treatment. Chief Occupational Therapists were assigned to the exhibits to provide the demonstrations and to carefully explain how the arts and craft activities were selected for the patients and how the patients engaged in activities. Their explanations included how the activities were structured, adapted, and modified for patients depending on their abilities. The demonstrations included such activities as spinning flax, weaving of hand towels and other items, block printing, metal working, and rug making. The demonstration of making willow-ware generated great interest as the public learned that patients were involved in all aspects of making willow-ware including planting and harvesting of willow holts on State Hospital grounds. The public learned this activity provided a healthful, open-air occupation for patients; that patients took pride in products they made from willow; and that these functional products were often used in the hospital setting (Slagle, 1926). With limited budgets, many occupational therapy departments made use of waste (recycled) materials such as left-over cloth and yarn and empty tin cans. The public was also very interested use of waste material to create beautiful craft objects and gave high praise to these objects (Slagle, 1927).

In addition to the display of the artistic handiworks, the department used visual aids such as wall charts explaining the purpose and value of different forms of treatment or growth of the occupational therapy department through the years. The exhibit continued to draw larger crowds each year with many return visitors. It proved to be an excellent public relations opportunity and a way to educate the public at large on occupational therapy in treatment of patients in the state institutions. Boy Scouts, Girl Scouts, 4-H children, teachers, and

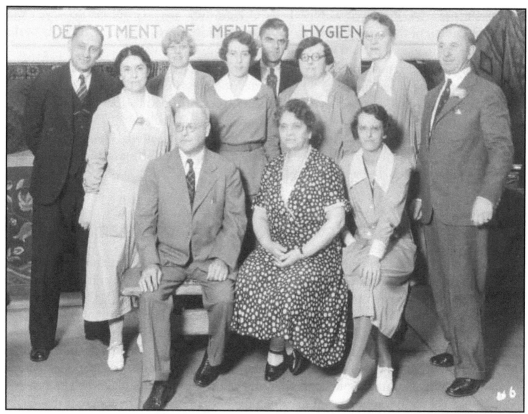

Figure 5-2. Representatives of the New York State Department of Mental Hygiene pictured at the 1931 New York State Fair. Mrs. Eleanor Clarke Slagle is sitting in the center of the first row. (Reprinted with permission of the Archive of the American Occupational Therapy Association, Inc.)

members of rural women's group visited the occupational therapy exhibit with great interest, and returned year after year. Other exhibitors were so enthusiastic about the occupational therapy exhibit that they often directed visitors to see the occupational therapy exhibit, and in some cases, physically guided visitors there. Sitting New York State governors, Governor Al Smith in 1927 and Governor Franklin D. Roosevelt in 1931, showed great interest in the exhibits and commended the Occupational Therapists overseeing the exhibit for the high quality of the goods displayed and the good work done in the State Hospitals (Slagle, 1929, 1933, 1934b). Mrs. Sara Delano Roosevelt, mother of Franklin D. Roosevelt, visited the occupational therapy exhibit at the State Fair in 1929 expressing interest in the development of the occupational therapy program and admiration for the quality of the products made by the patients (Slagle, 1931). Mrs. Eleanor Roosevelt visited the exhibit in 1930 and was particularly interested in the use of handicrafts as treatment (Slagle, 1932). The size of the occupational therapy exhibit, a booth 16 feet by 44 feet, was a measure of its success (Department of Mental Hygiene, 1935) (Figures 5-2 and 5-3). The occupational therapy department also displayed patient-made products in the Department of Mental Hygiene's booth during the 1939 New York World's Fair (Department of Mental Hygiene, 1941). And, following Mrs. Slagle's lead of promoting occupational therapy at fairs, Hudson River State Hospital displayed, and sold, patient made products at the Dutchess County Fair (Galante et al., 2018, p. 116).

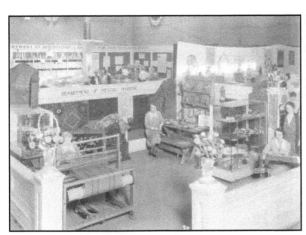

Figure 5-3. Occupational therapy exhibit at the 1931 New York State Fair. Mrs. Eleanor Clarke Slagle is standing at the right side of the photo. (Reprinted with permission of the Archive of the American Occupational Therapy Association, Inc.)

INTERNATIONAL PRESENTATIONS

The international recognition that the state's occupational therapy program received prompted the President of the Royal Medico-Psychological Society in England to invite Mrs. Slagle to present the program specifics to the Society. Mrs. Slagle set sail for England on the S.S. Champlain on Saturday, June 23, 1934. She arrived in Plymouth, England a week later on June 30, 1934 and proceeded to Northhampton, England to deliver her address ("Civic Club Met at New Hobart", 1934; "To Lecture in England", 1934; Slagle, 1936a). Her address, supplemented with exhibits, explained the organization of the New York State Department of Mental Hygiene, the locations and populations of the State institutions, and the different aspects and stages of the occupational therapy program outlined in her original plan. Mrs. Slagle also spoke about the records and forms used by the program, as well as the successful habit training program, the *Syllabus for Training of Nurses in Occupational Therapy,* and the *Game and Field Day Programs* (Exhibits - Office, E. C. S., Slagle, 1933, 1934c).

The National Council for Mental Hygiene in England also heard of Mrs. Slagle's successful occupational therapy programs. Invited by Sir Maurice Craig to address the Council after her address to Royal Medico-Psychological Society, Mrs. Slagle proceeded to London, England. There she spoke to the audience about occupational therapy and the recent advances in methods of treatment in America. Her next stop was to the famous Colony of Gheel in Belgium. The director of the colony, Dr. Sano, had invited Mrs. Slagle to learn about the methods used to treat patients with mental illness who live in the Colony of Gheel ("Civic Club Met at New Hobart", 1934; "To Lecture in England", 1934; Slagle, 1934a, 1936a). In the Colony of Gheel, rather than living in institutions, patients lived in private homes and moved freely around the community. After this enlightening visit, Mrs. Slagle boarded the S.S. Pennland in Antwerp on July 27, 1934, arriving home in Port of New York on August 6, 1934.

SUCCESSFUL PROGRAM EXPANSION

Mrs. Slagle greatly expanded the occupational therapy services in the first four years of her work with the New York State Hospital Commission (July 1, 1922 to June 30, 1926). The number of patients who participated in occupational therapy classes statewide went from 1,800 to 11,379 during these four years ("Good Work of Mrs. Slagle", 1927; Slagle, 1927). The staff of the occupational therapy department continued to grow year after year, with more and more patients receiving occupational therapy services. In 1927, the Bureau of Occupational Therapy employed 51 Occupational Therapists including those serving in administrative, supervisory, and staff capacities. By 1940, there were 71 Occupational Therapists employed in various capacities. Counting all the additional support staff, the number of employees in the Department totaled 126 in 1927 and 326 in 1940 (Department of Mental Hygiene, 1928b; Slagle, 1941). A total of 54,785 patients received therapy services in the last fiscal year that Mrs. Slagle served as the Director of Occupational Therapy (July 1941 to June 1942;

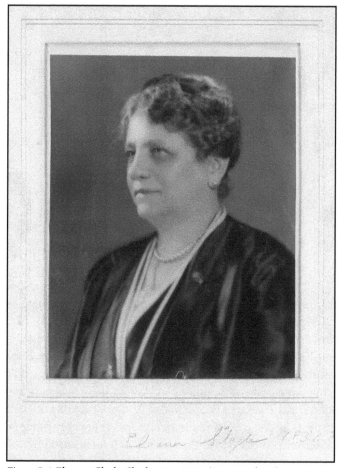

Figure 5-4. Eleanor Clarke Slagle circa 1936. (Reprinted with permission from the Research Library at the Fenimore Art Museum, Cooperstown, New York, John Davenport Clarke Papers, Coll. No. 12, Box 9, MWC.)

Department of Mental Hygiene, 1943b). The number of institutions and state schools in which occupational therapy was provided grew from 13 at the start of Mrs. Slagle's tenure to 26 (Slagle, 1936b) (Figure 5-4 and see Table 5-1). The benefit of the occupational therapy programs in the State Hospitals was recognized by one of the superintendents who stated, "Since the establishment of a regular, organized program of occupational therapy, there has come an indefinable change in our hospitals. It may not be, or is not, tangible, but it is certainly recognized by all concerned" (Slagle, 1931, p. 121).

REFLECTIONS ON THE PAST AND HOPES FOR THE FUTURE

By 1940, Mrs. Slagle was in her 70s and her health was failing. Despite this, she continued to work for the Department of Mental Hygiene. In the last few Bureau of Occupational Therapy reports that she submitted, she reflected on her years of work with the Department of Mental Hygiene. Looking back on her visionary plan, she admitted that initially there was some resistance to the changes required of the new programming. Giving great credit to the support and cooperation of the commissioners, superintendents, medical staff and employees, and especially to the efforts of the occupational therapy employees, she took great pride in the significant progress that had been made to achieving her vision (Slagle, 1941). Knowing that her tenure would come to an end in the next few years, her thoughts turned to making recommendations for the future including the need to continue research in occupational therapy, the need to cooperate with New York University and Columbia University occupational therapy programs, and the need to maintain high standards for occupational therapists (Slagle, 1942).

Anticipating the coming of the Second World War, the United States started to prepare for war. Mrs. Slagle suggested the department should compile data on Occupational Therapists employed by the State who could be called to service (Slagle, 1941). While not dismissing this suggestion, the Surgeon General's office projected the need for 30 Occupational Therapists which, the Surgeon General's office believed, could easily be provided by the American Red Cross (National Defense Committee, 1941; Slagle, 1942). To promote the need of highly trained Occupational Therapists in the war effort, Mrs. Slagle recounted the successful work of Occupational Therapists in World War I who stood up to meet the societal need of the time, reconstructing disabled military men (Slagle, 1943). Signing off on what was her last report to the Department of Mental Hygiene, she applauded the efforts to advance the care and understanding of patients with mental illness achieved by the professional teams of psychiatrists, nurses, social workers, and occupational therapists. Saluting all the occupational therapists, she finished her report writing, "It is to the last in this professional group of workers that we can and do hereby pay tribute" (Slagle, 1943, p. 133).

Well-known for the successful occupational therapy programs she established, such as the habit training program at the Phipps Psychiatric Clinic in Baltimore, the Community Workshop and the Henry B. Favill School in Chicago, and her work for the Illinois Department of Public Welfare (among other programs that she started and/or supervised), Mrs. Slagle was highly recruited by the top officials at the State Hospital Commission of New York. She did not disappoint them. As a result of her devoted and tireless efforts, Mrs. Slagle developed a premier occupational therapy department for New York State's Department of Mental Hygiene and, as Dr. Horatio Pollock had hoped years ago, "put New York more decidedly on the map" (AOTA, 1923).

She was an effective leader who initially worked against resistance to change a system to provide beneficial services to patients in state institutions. Step by step, she built an internationally recognized occupational therapy program to achieve her vision of a continuum of occupational therapy services in the New York State institutions. She recruited highly qualified individuals to organize, supervise, and provide occupational therapy services, and secured space, equipment, and supplies so they could implement the programs. She mentored her staff, instilling in them a sense of pride in their work, a hope for the future, a desire for lifelong learning, and the aspiration to improve occupational therapy methods. She educated physicians, nurses, and other health care practitioners—the professionals whose support she sought to expand occupational therapy programs. She willingly shared information with others, locally, nationally, and internationally, who wanted to establish similar types of occupational therapy programs. She promoted occupational therapy through public presentations, articles, pamphlets, the New York State Fair exhibits, and the 1939 New York World's Fair exhibit, all which carefully conveyed the purpose and distinct value of occupational therapy to the public. A true visionary leader, she succeeded in all these endeavors.

REFERENCES

Anderson, A. S. (1931, June 24). Patients have annual field day at Rochester State Hospital. *Democrat and Chronicle*, p. 15. Retrieved from www.newspapers.com

Annual Institute of Occupational Therapists. (1930). Psychiatric Quarterly, 4(3), 520-521. https://doi.org/10.1007/BF01579060AOTA. (1923). The sixth annual meeting of the American Occupational Therapy Association—Fourth day, Morning session. *Archives of the American Occupational Therapy Association, 2*(4), 309-328.

AOTA. (1924). The seventh annual meeting of the American Occupational Therapy Association. *Archives of Occupational Therapy, 3*(3), 235-245.

Civic Club Met at New Hobart. (1934, December 6). Civic club met at New Hobart: Mrs. Slagle was speaker on Tuesday afternoon. *Stamford Mirror Recorder*, p. 8. Retrieved from www.fultonhistory.com

Clarke, J. D. (1928, May 7). *[Letter to E. C. Slagle]*. Research Library at the Fenimore Art Museum (Collection 12, Box 4, Folder 16), Cooperstown, NY.

Cromwell, F. S. (1977). Eleanor Clarke Slagle, the leader, the woman. *The American Journal of Occupational Therapy, 31*(10), 645-648.

Department of Mental Hygiene. (1928a). To the Legislature of the State of New York. In *Thirty-Ninth Annual Report of the Department of Mental Hygiene* (p. 7). J. B. Lyon Company, Printers.

Department of Mental Hygiene. (1928b). Occupational therapy. In *Thirty-Ninth Annual Report of the Department of Mental Hygiene* (p. 52). J. B. Lyon Company, Printers.

Department of Mental Hygiene. (1931). Annual Institute of chief occupational therapists. In *Forty-Second Annual Report of the Department of Mental Hygiene* (pp. 64-66). J. B. Lyon Company, Printers.

Department of Mental Hygiene. (1934). Annual Institute of chief occupational therapists. In *Forty-Fifth Annual Report of the Department of Mental Hygiene* (pp. 74-75). J. B. Lyon Company, Printers.

Department of Mental Hygiene. (1935). Department exhibit at the State Fair. In *Forty-Sixth Annual Report of the Department of Mental Hygiene* (p. 78). J. B. Lyon Company, Printers.

Department of Mental Hygiene. (1941). World's Fair exhibit. In *Fifty-Second Annual Report of the Department of Mental Hygiene* (pp. 69-70). Department of Mental Hygiene.

Department of Mental Hygiene. (1943a). Annual Institute for Chief occupational therapists. In *Fifty-Fourth Annual Report of the Department of Mental Hygiene* (pp. 129-131). Department of Mental Hygiene.

Department of Mental Hygiene. (1943b). Occupational therapy. In *Fifty-Fourth Annual Report of the Department of Mental Hygiene* (p. 67). Department of Mental Hygiene.

Exhibits - Office, E. C. S., Slagle. (1933). *Draft of Presentation to the Royal Medico-Psychological Association.* Available from the Archive of the American Occupational Therapy Association, Bethesda, MD.

Fourth of July celebrated at State Hospital. (1932, July 7). *Gowanda Enterprise*, p. 1. Retrieved from www.fultonhistory.com

Galante, J., Rightmyer, L., & Hudson River State Hospital Nurses Alumni Association. (2018). *Hudson River State Hospital.* Arcadia Publishing.

Good work of Mrs. Slagle. (1927, April 8). *Oneonta Star*, p. 4. Retrieved from www.newspapers.com

Hospital here to have field day on June 7. (1934, May 17). *Utica Observer Dispatch*, p. 22. Retrieved from www.fultonhistory.com

Marcy Field Day Viewed by 2,200. (1935, June 5). *Daily Sentinel*, p. 1 (Second Section). Retrieved from www.fultonhistory.com

National Defense Committee. (1941, August 31). *Minutes of the meeting of the National Defense Committee of the American Occupational Therapy Association, August 31, 1941.* Archives of the American Occupational Therapy Association (Series 5, Box 25, Folder 169), Bethesda, MD.

New York State. (2020). *State fair history.* The fair: The great New York State Fair. Retrieved from https://nysfair.ny.gov/about/fair-history/

Occupational Therapy Notes. (1925, August). *Occupational Therapy and Rehabilitation, 4*(4), 297-302.

Slagle, E. C. (1921). Organizing an "O.T." Department. *Hospital Management, 12*(4), 43-45, 80.

Slagle, E. C. (1924). Report of the director of occupational therapy. In *Thirty-Fifth Annual Report of the State Hospital Commission* (pp. 71- 77). J. B. Lyon Company, Printers.

Slagle, E. C. (1925). Report of the director of occupational therapy. In *Thirty-Sixth Annual Report of the State Hospital Committee* (pp. 80-86). J. B. Lyon Company, Printers.

Slagle, E. C. (1926). Report of the director of occupational therapy. In *Thirty-Seventh Annual Report of the State Hospital Commission* (pp. 92- 99). J. B. Lyon Company, Printers.

Slagle, E. C. (1927). Report of director of occupational therapy. In *Thirty-Eighth Annual Report of the Department of Mental Hygiene* (pp. 80-87). J. B. Lyon Company, Printers.

Slagle, E. C. (1928). Report of director of occupational therapy. In *Thirty-Ninth Annual Report of the Department of Mental Hygiene* (pp. 94-99). J. B. Lyon Company, Printers.

Slagle, E. C. (1929). Report of the Bureau of Occupational Therapy. In *Fortieth Annual Report of the Department of Mental Hygiene* (pp. 108-115). J. B. Lyon Company, Printers.

Slagle, E. C. (1930). Annual report of the Bureau of Occupational Therapy. In *Forty-First Annual Report of the Department of Mental Hygiene* (pp. 113-121). J. B. Lyon Company, Printers.

Slagle, E. C. (1931). Report of the Director of the Bureau of Occupational Therapy. In *Forty-Second Annual Report of the Department of Mental Hygiene* (pp. 115-123). J. B. Lyon Company, Printers.

Slagle, E. C. (1932). Report of the Director of the Bureau of Occupational Therapy. In *Forty-Second Annual Report of the Department of Mental Hygiene* (pp. 131-139). Burland Printing Company, Inc.

Slagle, E. C. (1933). Report of the Bureau of Occupational Therapy. In *Forty-Fourth Annual Report of the Department of Mental Hygiene* (pp. 137-145). J. B. Lyon Company, Printers.

Slagle, E. C. (1934a). Occupational therapy: Recent methods and advances in the United States. *Occupational Therapy & Rehabilitation, 13*(5), 289-298.

Slagle, E. C. (1934b). Report of the Bureau of Occupational Therapy. In *Forty-Fifth Annual Report of the Department of Mental Hygiene* (pp. 135-145). J. B. Lyon Company, Printers.

Slagle, E. C. (1934c). The occupational therapy programme in the State of New York. *British Journal of Psychiatry (Journal of Mental Science), 80,* 639-649.

Slagle, E. C. (1935). Report of the Bureau of Occupational Therapy. In *Forty-Sixth Annual Report of the Department of Mental Hygiene* (pp. 130-141). J. B. Lyon Company, Printers.

Slagle, E. C. (1936a). Report of the Bureau of Occupational Therapy. In *Forty-Seventh Annual Report of the Department of Mental Hygiene* (pp. 130-141). J. B. Lyon Company, Printers.

Slagle, E. C. (1936b). The past, present, and future of occupational therapy in the State Department of Mental Hygiene. *Psychiatric Quarterly, 10*(1), 144-156.

Slagle, E. C. (1937). Report of the Bureau of Occupational Therapy. In *Forty-Eighth Annual Report of the Department of Mental Hygiene* (pp. 135-145). J. B. Lyon Company, Printers.

Slagle, E. C. (1938). Report of the Bureau of Occupational Therapy. In *Forty-Ninth Annual Report of the Department of Mental Hygiene* (pp. 115-123). J. B. Lyon Company, Printers.

Slagle, E. C. (1940). Report of the Bureau of Occupational Therapy. In *Fifty-First Annual Report of the Department of Mental Hygiene* (pp. 125-136). J. B. Lyon Company, Printers.

Slagle, E. C. (1941). Report of the Bureau of Occupational Therapy. In *Fifty-Second Annual Report of the Department of Mental Hygiene* (pp. 126-136). Department of Mental Hygiene.

Slagle, E. C. (1942). Report of the Bureau of Occupational Therapy. In *Fifty-Third Annual Report of the Department of Mental Hygiene* (pp. 136-144). Department of Mental Hygiene.

Slagle, E. C. (1943). Report of the Bureau of Occupational Therapy. In *Fifty-Fourth Annual Report of the Department of Mental Hygiene* (pp. 125-133). Department of Mental Hygiene.

Slagle, E. C., & Robeson, H. A. (1941). *Syllabus for training of nurses in occupational therapy* (2nd ed.). State Hospitals Press.

State Hospital Commission. (1925a). The bond issue campaign (pp. 20-25). In *Thirty-Sixth Annual Report of the State Hospital Committee.* J. B. Lyon Company, Printers.

State Hospital Commission. (1925b). Institute in occupational therapy. In *Thirty-Sixth Annual Report of the State Hospital Committee* (p. 41). J. B. Lyon Company, Printers.

The State Hospital Quarterly. (1922, August). News and comment: New Items. *The State Hospital Quarterly, 7*(4), 656 - 660.

To Lecture in England. (1934, July 5). *Windham Journal,* p. 1. Retrieved from www.fultonhistory.com

LIFE'S HONORS
AND LEGACIES

> *"The integrity of your profession is in your hands.*
> *I bid you all Godspeed in your work."*
> Eleanor Clarke Slagle (1937a, p. 345)

On January 2, 1937, after 20 years of dedicated volunteer service to the AOTA, Mrs. Slagle submitted a letter to Dr. Joseph C. Doane, President of the AOTA, resigning her position as Secretary-Treasurer (Slagle, 1937b, January 2). Later that year, in tribute to her lengthy service, on the morning of September 14, 1937 at the Annual AOTA Conference in Atlantic City, New Jersey, Mrs. Slagle was made an Honorary President of the AOTA (AOTA, 1937a). That evening, a Testimonial Dinner was held in her honor at the Hotel Chelsea (AOTA, 1937b). Mrs. Eleanor Roosevelt, wife of President Franklin D. Roosevelt and First Lady of the United States, attended the dinner and paid tribute to Mrs. Slagle during the ceremonies. Not only did Mrs. Roosevelt speak at the event, she wrote about this occasion in her "My Day" syndicated newspaper article, touting the benefits of occupational therapy to the nation (Roosevelt, 1937; The Associated Press, 1937) (Figure 6-1).

At the dinner, on behalf of a grateful membership of the AOTA, Dr. Doane presented Mrs. Slagle with "a gift of money in a container"—a check for $2000, quite a substantial amount in 1937. The gift was inscribed:

> Eleanor Clarke Slagle—She has been the corner stone in the development and promotion of occupational therapy. Now we in turn ask that she accept our gift as the corner stone of her new home which we hope will be the place of rest and happiness and release from the arduous duties. We offer it with deep affection and profound gratitude for her twenty-one years of untiring service in our behalf. (Pollock, 1942)

Mrs. Slagle was 46 years old when she attended the Inaugural Meeting in Clifton Springs, New York in 1917. She was 66 years of age when she resigned her volunteer position with the AOTA. She was indeed proud of her 20 years of tireless service, first as a founder of the association and then as an officer guiding the development of the association and the profession of occupational therapy. Acknowledging that it was time for others to take up the work and conquer the new frontiers, speaking from the heart Mrs. Slagle borrowed a quote from George Edward Barton, the first president of the National Society for the Promotion of Occupational Therapy/American Occupational Therapy Association, "I relinquish the honour of being your officer, proud to have been of any assistance to a cause so noble, and I lay down the office content in the knowledge that it can be more ably filled". Further, Mrs. Slagle encouraged others to continue the good work with the message, "The integrity of your profession is in your hands. I bid you all Godspeed in your work" (Slagle, 1937a, p. 345).

TRIBUTES

Miss Harriet A. Robeson, one of Mrs. Slagle's long time friends and colleagues, was in a unique position to characterize and give insight into Mrs. Slagle's years of work for the profession. Miss Robeson had worked closely with Mrs. Slagle in her capacities as Director of Occupational Therapy at King's Park State Hospital

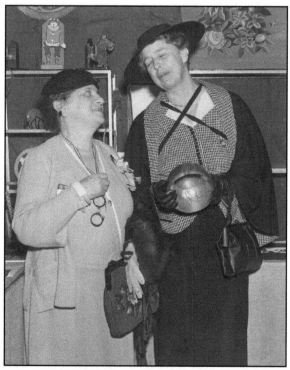

Figure 6-1. Eleanor Clarke Slagle (left) and Eleanor Roosevelt, First Lady of the United States (right) admiring a product made by a patient in occupational therapy. (Reprinted with permission from the Research Library at the Fenimore Art Museum, Cooperstown, New York, John Davenport Clarke Papers, Coll. No. 12, Box 9, MWC.)

for the New York State Hospital Commission, Assistant Director of Occupational Therapy for the New York State Department of Mental Hygiene, co-author with Mrs. Slagle of *Syllabus for Training of Nurses in Occupational Therapy,* and as a long time member of the AOTA's Board of Management ("Our Writers", 1937). In the 1937 edition of the *Journal of Occupational Therapy,* the only edition ever published, Miss Robeson gave a thoughtful, heartfelt tribute full of admiration for Mrs. Slagle. Miss Robeson portrayed the many roles Mrs. Slagle filled, her activities, and her trials and tribulations, writing:

> Imagine the duties of President, Treasurer, Executive Secretary, Specialist, Travelling Salesman, Promotor, Advocate, and Ghost Writer combined into one job, and that would be but a part of the picture of the office Mrs. Slagle has filled these past twenty years in the AOTA. (Robeson, 1937, p. 3)

In addressing Mrs. Slagle's efforts to develop and update minimum standards of training for Occupational Therapists and to establish a national directory that lists qualified Occupational Therapists, Miss Robeson wrote:

> [these were] momentous steps, but in no way can they tell of the years of study, consultation, planning, testing, adapting, until each step became feasible and the final accomplishment possible. Mrs. Slagle has directed and laid the foundation stones on which our profession and our national organization rest today. (Robeson, 1937, p. 4)

Speaking to Mrs. Slagle's steadfastness in advancing the profession, Miss Robeson wrote:

> Those of us who have been privileged to follow the winding trail of these years know of struggles, of courage in facing criticism, of disappointments and rewards; the patient waiting, persistent faith, personal troubles and sorrows ignored; the sapping of vitality and health—all that the sick of the world might benefit by a sound program of occupational treatment and that it might be administered by highly qualified personnel. (Robeson, 1937, p. 4)

A presiding official at the 1930 AOTA Conference in New Orleans recognizing the tireless work of Eleanor Clarke Slagle predicted the future, stating that because of her sustained efforts her name would stand out in history. This prediction proved true as her name and place in history was firmly established with the creation of the Eleanor Clarke Slagle Lectureship, so named to honor her substantial contributions to the profession ("Former Hobart Girl Honored", 1931). To recognize and honor the many tributes paid to Mrs. Slagle, the Eleanor Clarke Slagle Lectureship was created by a vote in the House of Delegates and Board of Managers of the AOTA in 1953 to recognize selected AOTA members' meritorious service to the profession (AOTA, 1954). Now considered one of the highest awards bestowed by AOTA, the "purpose is to honor a member of the Association who has substantially and innovatively contributed to the development of the body of knowledge of the profession through research, education, and/or clinical practice" (AOTA, 2019a).

FINAL YEARS

In the spring of 1939, after a search for her perfect country house, she settled on a house on Farrington Avenue in Philipse Manor, North Tarrytown, New York. The generous gift given to her by the membership of the AOTA was, in part, used to purchase this house in Westchester County. The house was conveniently located a few blocks from the Philipse Manor Train Station, a station on the Hudson Line on the east side of the Hudson River. The proximity of this station to her new house allowed her to take the train to her New York City office for her work with the New York State Department of Mental Hygiene.

In later life she suffered from sciatica and arteriosclerosis (Bing, 1997). In early 1940, while getting ready for a trip to Florida, she slipped on a rug and injured her back. For a time she was required to wear a plastic jacket, limiting some of her activities. Despite her condition, she continued to work at home, traveling to her office once a week to meet with her secretary and conduct business. Mrs. Slagle's many friends were concerned about the physical strain of her work schedule, especially since "she had had a weak heart for at least 10 years" (Editorial, 1942, p. 374). Despite her poor health, Mrs. Slagle continued her work for the New York State Department of Mental Hygiene and maintained an active interest and contributed to the profession until her death in September 1942 (Editorial, 1942) (Figure 6-2).

In the late 1930s and early 1940s, Mrs. Slagle began to exchange letters with Beatrice Wade, an Occupational Therapist from Illinois and future leader of the profession. These letters, found in the Archive of the AOTA, demonstrate Mrs. Slagle's continued interest in the profession. The correspondence covered a number of topics, including upcoming conferences and round table discussions, the status of the Illinois Department of Public Hygiene and Illinois State institutional affairs, as well as discussions about various people they knew. On September 11, 1942, Mrs. Slagle wrote to Ms. Wade inquiring about a planned meeting of

the AOTA executives scheduled to be held in New York
City in October. As Ms.
Wade was a member of the
Board of Management, Mrs.
Slagle presumed that Ms.
Wade would be attending
the meeting and expressed
the hope to see her when she
came to New York (Slagle,
1942). They did not meet in
New York. Mrs. Slagle died
on September 18, 1942, one
week after writing that letter
to Ms. Wade. Mrs. Slagle's
many friends and profes-
sional colleagues mourned
her passing.

FUNERAL SERVICES

Funeral services for
Mrs. Slagle were held on
September 21, 1942 in the
historic Christ Episcopal
Church in Tarrytown, New
York. In compliance with
her wishes, simple Episcopal
rites were performed and no
eulogy was delivered. Given

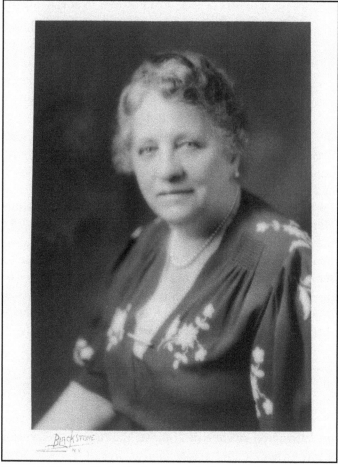

Figure 6-2. Eleanor Clarke Slagle in later life. (Reprinted with permission from the Research Library at the Fenimore Art Museum, Cooperstown, New York, John Davenport Clarke Papers, Coll. No. 12, Box 7.)

her position and lengthy service to the State Department of Mental Hygiene numerous dig-
nitaries were present for the funeral, many serving as honorary pallbearers. Dr. William G.
Tiffany, Commissioner of the State Department of Mental Hygiene, and Dr. Frederick W.
Parsons, his predecessor, were among the notables attending. After the service, Mrs. Slagle's
body was transported by hearse to Hobart, New York for burial in the Clarke Family plot in
Locust Hill Cemetery, a peaceful setting less than a mile from where she was born ("Mrs.
Eleanor Slagle, State Aide, Mourned at Rites", 1942). Since then, Mrs. Slagle, once nationally
and internationally known, has rested in peace, and until now, relatively unknown to citizens
of her hometown of Hobart, New York (Figures 6-3 and 6-4).

The New York State Department of Mental Hygiene paid tribute to Mrs. Slagle, including
her obituary in the 1942-1943 Annual Report (Department of Mental Hygiene, 1944)—an
honor accorded to those who held high level positions with the State. Dr. Horatio M. Pollock,
Director of Mental Hygiene Statistics for the New York State Department of Mental Hygiene
(who worked closely with Mrs. Slagle to develop forms for records and reports in order to
maintain statistics for the Bureau of Occupational Therapy) in tribute published an article,

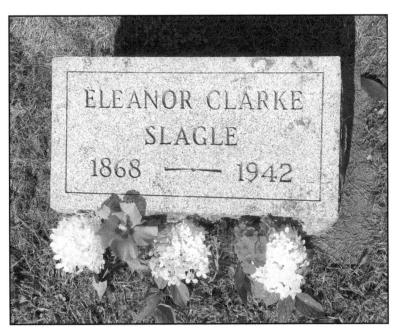

Figure 6-3. Eleanor Clarke Slagle's headstone in Locust Hill Cemetery. (© Lori T. Andersen. Reprinted with permission.)

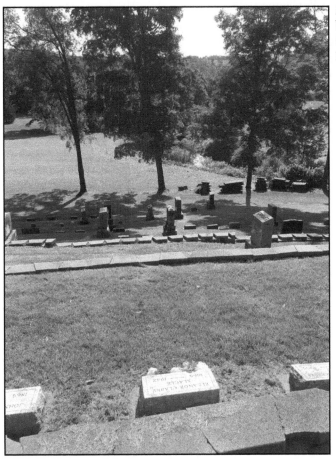

Figure 6-4. Eleanor Clarke Slagle's burial place overlooking Town Brook. (© Lori T. Andersen. Reprinted with permission.)

Biographical Sketch of Eleanor Clarke Slagle, in the November 1942 issue of the *American Journal of Psychiatry* (Pollock, 1942). In 1946, Mrs. Virginia Scullin, previously Chief Occupational Therapist at Pilgrim State Hospital, was appointed Director of Occupational Therapy as Mrs. Slagle's successor (Department of Mental Hygiene, 1947; "Director Named for Nurse Unit", 1946).

GROWTH OF THE PROFESSION

In 1923 at the Seventh Annual Meeting of AOTA, while reminiscing about the late Dr. Herbert J. Hall, fourth president of the AOTA, Mrs. Slagle shared that the fun-loving Dr. Hall referred to her as the "The Grandmother of the Revolution" (AOTA, 1924, p. 152). It was a revolution indeed, a revolution that brought about significant change ... a revolution that improved the quality of life for so many.

Much had changed since the establishment of the National Society for the Promotion of Occupational Therapy/American Occupational Therapy Association in March 1917. Six people attended the first meeting held at Consolation House in Clifton Springs, New York. More than 14,000 people attended the Centennial Conference held in March 2017 in Philadelphia, Pennsylvania. Membership in the society grew from six people in 1917, to more than 60,000 in 2017, the year that marked AOTA's Centennial Celebration. In 2019, it was reported that the Accreditation Council for Occupational Therapy Education (ACOTE), now "accredits or is in the process of accrediting over 570 occupational therapy and occupational therapy assistant educational programs in the United States and its territories as well as programs in the United Kingdom" (AOTA, 2019b). In the summer of 2019, there were more than 183,000 certified occupational therapy practitioners including 130,254 certified occupational therapists and 52,914 certified occupational therapy assistants who met educational standards set by the National Board for Certification of Occupational Therapists (National Board for Certification of Occupational Therapy, 2019).

In 2020, in Mrs. Slagle's home state of New York where she wanted to establish an occupational therapy school, there were 34 accredited schools—22 schools that educate occupational therapists and 12 schools that educate occupational therapy assistants (Accreditation Council for Occupational Therapy Education, 2020). As of January 1, 2020, more than 19,900 occupational therapy practitioners were licensed by New York State (New York State Education Department, 2020).

In her volunteer work with the AOTA, Mrs. Slagle was able to work with others to establish high standards for the education of Occupational Therapists to ensure their ability to provide high quality occupational therapy services. In her work with the New York State Department of Mental Hygiene, she was able to educate health care practitioners and the public about the distinct value of occupational therapy—bringing increased awareness and recognition to the new profession. Mrs. Slagle was able to point to the successes of these programs implemented by the highly qualified staff under her supervision to expand the occupational therapy program statewide, and to promote the development of other occupational therapy programs statewide, nationally, and internationally. Much of this was accomplished through the shear force of her personality, professionalism, political awareness, and desire to help others. As such, "Mother of Occupational Therapy" and "Grandmother of the Revolution" are both fitting titles for the woman so instrumental in building a strong foundation for the AOTA; promoting the profession of occupational therapy, nationally and internationally; and developing a premier occupational therapy program in New York State. The profession of occupational therapy stands on the shoulders of this giant among giants and honors her exceptional service and accomplishments.

REFERENCES

Accreditation Council for Occupational Therapy Education. (2020). *School Directory—New York State Accredited Schools.* https://acoteonline.org/schools/?cn-cat-in%5B%5D=&cn-cat-in%5B%5D=&cn-cat-in%5B%5D=15&cn-region=NY

AOTA. (1924). Seventh Annual Meeting of the American Occupational Therapy Association: Tuesday, October 30, 1923, Afternoon Session. *Archives of Occupational Therapy, 3*(2), 145-159.

AOTA. (1937a). Twenty-First Annual Meeting of the American Occupational Therapy Association. *Occupational Therapy and Rehabilitation, 16*(5), 335-341.

AOTA. (1937b). *Program: Twenty-first annual meeting, Atlantic City, N. J., September 13, 14, 15, 16, 1937.* Archive of the American Occupational Therapy Association (Series 8, Folder 460, Box 64), Bethesda, MD.

AOTA. (1954). Annual reports: Meeting of the House of Delegates. *American Journal of Occupational Therapy, 8*(1), 24-35.

AOTA. (2019b). *Accreditation.* Retrieved from https://www.aota.org/Education-Careers/Accreditation.aspx

AOTA. (2019a). *Award descriptions.* Retrieved from https://www.aota.org/Education-Careers/Awards/descriptions.aspx

Bing, R. K. (1997). "And teach agony to sing": An afternoon with Eleanor Clarke Slagle. *The American Journal of Occupational Therapy, 51*(3), 220-227.

Department of Mental Hygiene. (1944). Death of Mrs. Eleanor Clarke Slagle. In *Fifty-Fifth Annual Report of the Department of Mental Hygiene* (p. 14). Department of Mental Hygiene.

Department of Mental Hygiene. (1947). Other major appointments. In *Fifty-Eighth Annual Report of the Department of Mental Hygiene* (p. 21). Department of Mental Hygiene.

Director Named for Nurse Unit. (1946, June 9). *Utica Observer Dispatch*, p. 2. Retrieved from www.fultonhistory.com

Editorial. (1942). Eleanor Clarke Slagle memorial. *Occupational Therapy and Rehabilitation, 21*(5), 373-374.

Former Hobart girl honored. (1931). *Stamford Mirror-Recorder,* p. 8. Retrieved from www.fultonhistory.com

Mrs. Eleanor Slagle, State aide, mourned at rites. (1942, September 21). *The Daily News*, p. 1-2. Retrieved from www.fultonhistory.com

National Board for Certification of Occupational Therapy. (2019, Summer). Certificants by the numbers. *Certification Matters—Newsletter of the National Board for Certification of Occupational Therapy*, p. 4.

New York State Education Department. (2020). Occupational therapy license statistics. Retrieved from http://www.op.nysed.gov/prof/ot/otcounts.htmOur Writers. (1937). *Journal of Occupational Therapy*, 48.

Pollock, H. M. (1942). In Memoriam: Eleanor Clarke Slagle—1876-1942. *American Journal of Psychiatry, 99*(3), 472-474.

Robeson, H. A. (1937, September). Eleanor Clarke Slagle. *Journal of Occupational Therapy*, 3-4.

Roosevelt, E. (1937, September 16). My day. *Pittsburgh Press,* p. 27. Retrieved from www.newspapers.com

Slagle, E. C. (1937a). Editorial: From the heart. *Occupational Therapy and Rehabilitation, 16*(5), 343-345.

Slagle, E. C. (1937b, January 2). *[Letter to J. C. Doane].* Archive of the American Occupational Therapy Association (Series 5, Box 24, Folder 162), Bethesda, MD.

Slagle, E. C. (1942, September 11). *[Letter to Beatrice Wade].* Archive of the American Occupational Therapy Association (Included in Beatrice Wade's folder with transcript of oral interview), Bethesda, MD.

The Associated Press. (1937, September 16). Mrs. Roosevelt praises therapy: Urges it as occupation for persons needing emotional outlet: Lauds work of Ass'n. *Gazette and Daily*, p. 4. Retrieved from www.newspapers.com

CLARK(E) FAMILY TREE

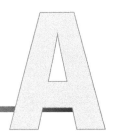

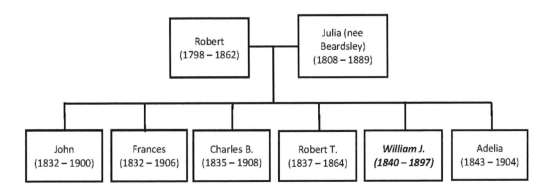

The Clark family tree with Eleanor Clarke Slagle's paternal grandparents; her father, William; and her aunts and uncles.

Note: There are inconsistencies in census records and military records, so it is possible that John and Frances were born in 1832 and 1833 respectively.

DAVENPORT FAMILY TREE

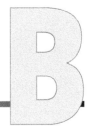

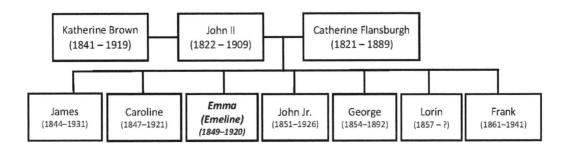

Davenport family tree with Eleanor Clarke Slagle's maternal grandparents; her mother, Emma; and her aunts and uncles.

LOCATION OF
CLARK FAMILY HOMESTEAD

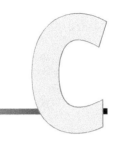

A number of buildings built in the mid 1800s to early 1900s, as well as open spaces, are part of the lot at 284 Main Street. This is the present site of Second Wind Furniture and Antiques, where the Clark(e) family homestead was located. The Clark house, a two-story building made of bricks, no longer stands on the lot today as it was destroyed by fire in 1941 ("Fire Damaged Hobart House", 1941; Meagley, 2014, p. 93). The precise location of the Clark house was confirmed by comparing maps of the area. The book, *Century of Hobart: 1888-1988,* identifies a house next to the Kermit and Margaret Cantwell house and the Cantwell Insurance Office as the birthplace of Congressman John D. Clarke (Hobart Historical Society, 1988, p. 31) (Figure C-1). That particular location is consistent with the 1869 Beers Map of the village of Hobart that shows a house at that location occupied by 'JClark' (Beers, 1869), a reference to Julia Clark or John Clark (Meagley, 2014, p. 93). Finally, the 1927 Sanborn Fire Insurance Map of Hobart, New York depicts a sketch of a two-story building at that location with a "U-shape" shading in the middle of the building. According to the key on the map, the shading on the sketch indicates that the house was partially constructed of brick (Sanborn Map Company, 1927), consistent with reports that the Clarke house was made of bricks. Arrows on a photo taken at the east end of the circular drive in front of Second Wind Furniture and Antiques and on a Google Earth map of the 284 Main Street lot mark the location of an old well. The presence of that old well suggests that a house once stood at that location (Figures C-2 and C-3).

The maps and photos shown in Figures C-1, C-2, and C-3 identify the following buildings/locations, which show a portion of Main Street (formerly named West Main Street) in Hobart, New York:

- A—The former Kermit and Margaret Cantwell House, now home to current owners of Second Wind Furniture and Antiques.
- B—Current location of Second Wind Furniture and Antiques, 284 Main Street, and previous location of the Cantwell Insurance Office.
- C—Location of an old well at the previous site of the Clark Family homestead, birthplace of John Davenport Clarke and Eleanor Clarke Slagle.

Figure C-1. Adapted from the book, *A Century of Hobart: 1888-1988* published by the Hobart Historical Society, 1988. (Reprinted with permission from the Hobart Historical Society, Hobart, NY.)

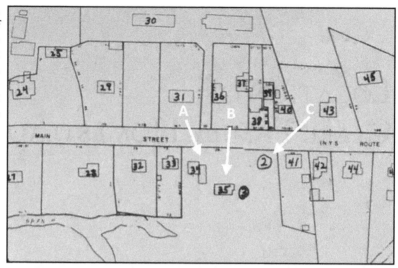

Figure C-2. Google Earth view of 284 Main Street. Adapted from Google Earth.

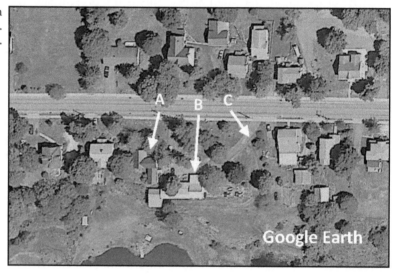

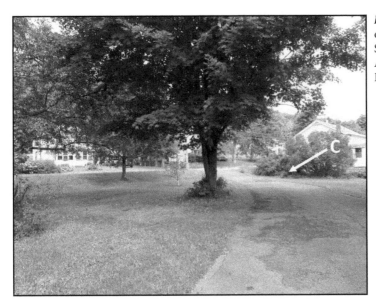

Figure C-3. Photo of the east end of the circular drive in front of Second Wind Furniture and Antiques. (© Lori T. Andersen. Reprinted with permission.)

REFERENCES

Beers, F. W. (1869). Bovina, Hobart. In *Atlas of Delaware County New York 1869.* F. W. Beers, A. D. Ellis, G. G. Soule.

Fire damaged Hobart house. (1941, January 9). *Stamford Mirror-Recorder,* p. 8. Available in Hobart Historical Society's Scrapbook #7.

Hobart Historical Society. (1988). *A century of Hobart, 1888-1988.* Hobart Historical Society.

Meagley, J. G. (2014). *A look back at Hobart, NY on the 125th Anniversary of the Village Incorporation, 1888-2013.* Hobart Historical Society.

Sanborn Map Company. (1927). *Sanborn fire insurance map from Hobart, Delaware County, New York.* Sanborn Map Company. Available at the Hobart Historical Society, Hobart, New York.

Locations in Hobart

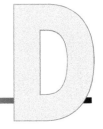

The locations of importance to Eleanor Clarke Slagle's life in the village of Hobart are all within walking distance. To help the reader visualize the area and relative distances, a map identifies locations of interest.

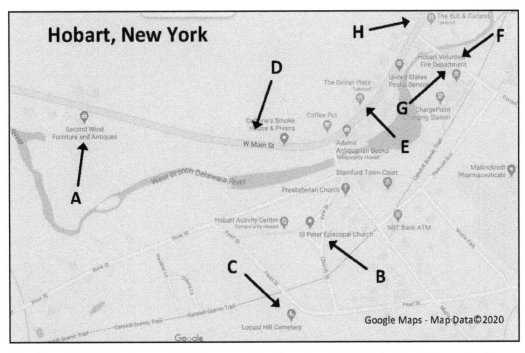

A – Second Wind Furniture and Antiques, previous location of the Clarke Family homestead.

B – St. Peter's Episcopal Church, location of the Clark-Slagle wedding in 1894.

C – Locust Hill Cemetery, resting place of Eleanor Clarke Slagle and members of her family.

D – Previous location of the William J. and Emma Clark's house, where Ella May Clark lived the first years of her life.

E – The Hobart Inn is located at the same location as the Dinner Plate, 645 Main Street. Known as Scutt's Hotel in the 1860s, it was the location where Robert Clark, Eleanor's grandfather, was fatally injured in a fight.

F – Location of the former home of St. Andrew's Masonic Lodge, No. 289, now home to the Hobart Historical Society.

G – Location of the former Grant's Opera House.

H – Location of the former New Hobart Hotel.

INDEX

CPSIA information can be obtained
at www.ICGtesting.com
Printed in the USA
LVHW020736250522
719533LV00005B/9